The Science of Everything

The Man Who Invented Email Reveals the
Science That Interconnects Everything

SYSTEMS HEALTH® SERIES

V.A. Shiva PhD

The Inventor of Email

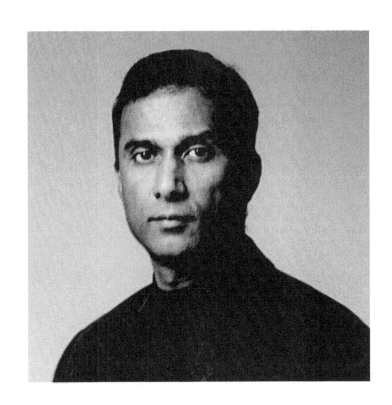

Dr. V. A. Shiva

To the Great Siddhars

Printed in the United States of America.

First Edition, 2016.

ISBN 978-0-9985049-1-9

General Interactive, LLC
Publishing Division
701 Concord Ave.
Cambridge, MA 02138
www.generalinteractive.com

All proceeds from the sale of this book go to Innovation Corps, a 501 (c) not-for-profit project.
www.innovation-corps.org

Contents

INTRODUCTION   7

PART 1: The Journey to Systems   13
   CHAPTER 1: A Child of Oppression and Truth   14
   CHAPTER 2: The Invention of Email   22
   CHAPTER 3: Somethings Need to Be Destroyed   29

PART 2: Systems Biology   39
   CHAPTER 4: Revolutionary Road   40
   CHAPTER 5: Beyond Reductionism   44
   CHAPTER 6: Systems of Systems   48
   CHAPTER 7: Modeling the Whole Cell   53

PART 3: The First Systems Biology   59
   CHAPTER 8: Siddha and Ayurveda   60
   CHAPTER 9: Layers of Meaning   66
   CHAPTER 10: Siddha's Model of a Human Being   70
   CHAPTER 11: The Architecture of Existence   73
   CHAPTER 12: Vata, Pitta, Kapha   77

PART 4: Systems Theory   83
   CHAPTER 13: The Systems Toolbox   84
   CHAPTER 14: Open Systems   88
   CHAPTER 15: Open Systems   91
   CHAPTER 16: An Intelligent System in Action   95
   CHAPTER 17: Systems Theory in the Kitchen   98

PART 5: The Rosetta Stone and Beyond   101
   CHAPTER 18: The Bridge Between Two Worlds   102
   CHAPTER 19: The Connective Tissue   106
   CHAPTER 20: Holism and Personalization   110

PART 6: The System of Your Physical Self   113
   CHAPTER 21: Your Body is an Intelligent System   114
   CHAPTER 22: Identifying Disturbances   119
   CHAPTER 23: Dealing With Disturbances   122

PART 7 The Science of Everything at the Movies   137
   CHAPTER 24: Gladiator   138
   CHAPTER 25: Apollo 13   143
   CHAPTER 26: Joy   148

INTRODUCTION

My journey to this book -- that is, to *The Science of Everything* -- began with a childhood passion for medicine.

That passion was originally inspired by watching my grandmother treat and heal people who lined up outside her home in Muhavur, a small village in South India. How did she do that? Where did she learn her skills? Could I learn them too?

Those questions led me on the long and winding path that I will revisit with you in these pages. Along that path, I earned four degrees at MIT in fields of engineering, architecture and biology. Then, disillusioned by the many problems I observed in conventional medicine, I studied various forms of traditional and alternative healthcare systems.

Still later, with the emergence of Systems Biology -- modern science's holistic approach to medicine -- my research in Systems Biology revealed connections across continents and centuries between modern systems theory, or more specifically control systems engineering, and the ancient healing science of Siddha.

In this connection I discovered the Science of Everything. In my research to integrate modern systems theory and ancient healing wisdom, I discovered the profound missing link between mind and body, and a common language that bridges the wisdom of East and West, ancient and modern, science and tradition. These discoveries are the foundations of this book, which will provide you a new understanding of what are the common principles that affect all systems in nature and reveal who you truly are.

When it comes to building a universal understanding of all things, "the theory of everything" is a phrase that comes up every once in awhile. You may have heard it in several different contexts. For instance, *The Theory of Everything* is the title of a film about the British physicist Stephen Hawking. The film stars Eddie Redmayne as the severely disabled scientist, and Felicity Jones as his wife. Eddie Redmayne won an Oscar for his role, and the film was also nominated for Best Picture.

The title of the film is also a reference to a problem in physics which has challenged Hawking, and has been a fundamental problem in science since the early 20th century. Albert Einstein was preoccupied with it for most of his later life.

Put very simply, the problem in physics involves integrating Einstein's theory of gravitation -- which describes space, time, and matter on the vast scale of the whole universe from planets to galaxies -- with quantum mechanics, which deals with the smallest possible scale of elementary particles. So far no one in physics has been able to describe or demonstrate the unity of the forces which traverse across these infinite spatial scales -- not Einstein, and not Stephen Hawking either.

But I have discovered "The Science of Everything," although I'm not a physicist. And, what I'm going to share with you reveals a common set of principles that affects all systems from the infinitesimal to the infinite.

In fact, not being a physicist is the reason I was able to make that discovery. I'm an engineer, and as an engineer, I'm not oriented toward decades of abstract speculation in a university. Engineers have to build things that work. Doing that requires a practical set of principles that can be universally applied.

That set of principles exists in modern systems theory, which began to emerge as a specific scientific field in the 1930s. Systems theory really can be applied to everything, as you'll learn in the chapters that follow. Systems theory is a powerful unifying tool through which literally anything can be understood -- anything from biology to economics to human history and, especially, human health.

As I studied systems theory at MIT and later applied it in my work, I made an astonishing discovery that is actually an extension of systems theory as a unifying force. I realized that the ancient Indian wisdom tradition called Siddha, developed more than 5,000 years ago, expresses a unifying perspective that modern systems theory is now replicating.

The foundations of Siddha, the world's first application of systems thinking, are the same as the foundations of today's Control Systems Engineering --- the engineering principles that are the foundation of nearly every major engineering development. The terminology may be different, but the results are the same. This is not just a *theory* of everything. It's a science and its practical application. In this book, you'll learn what those principles are and how to apply the Science of Everything to benefit your own life.

But who am I to have succeeded where Einstein and Hawking failed?

My personal background, detailed in Part One, *Journey to Systems*, provides a glimpse into the impetus for that success. From my birth, I was exposed to *systems* --- systems of oppression as well as systems of truth. My journey to understand the nature of those systems --- a journey in many ways motivated not by conscious choice --- is at the heart of my work as a scientist, inventor and revolutionary. I say revolutionary because my intent is to destroy those long-standing systems of oppression, and to create and rediscover those systems that bring truth, freedom and health. In my other books, I also include this Part as a core module of the content in order to provide you insights of how the path I traversed directly motivated my fascination with systems. If you've read it before, you can skip to Part Two.

Part Two will start in the West with my training in systems biology --- the end of a journey across those four degrees from MIT. You will be introduced to the principles of the emerging field of systems biology --- a new field which aims to address many of the problems with the reductionism of western biology. This will provide you the foundation to understand that the West's recent inspiration for a systems-based approach to biology is what others in the East traversed many millennia ago.

Part Three discusses the core principles of Siddha, which are revealed not only as an ancient wisdom tradition, but also as a striking and modern holistic model of our environment on every scale from the largest to the smallest, from the individual cell to the universe itself. This, you will learn, is truly "the first systems biology."

Part Four provides a detailed explanation of modern control systems engineering theory. This knowledge is what I learned at MIT. However, my attempt here is to bring this knowledge to you so you can easily understand and appreciate it, as well as its relevance, and how it operates in the physical world.

Part Five -- "The Rosetta Stone" -- reveals the fundamental link that I discovered during my Fulbright Research between the core principles of modern control systems engineering and the core principles of Siddha. This opens the door to the Science of Everything, at a time when Western science desperately needs to move beyond reductionism toward an engineering systems approach.

Part Six provides guidelines for self-identifying, using the Science of Everything, the interactions of systems elements in your own body, as well as tools for restoring health when those elements become unbalanced. Your body is the most easily accessible "laboratory" to see how the Science of Everything is in play all the time.

Finally, I've included Part Seven, where the Science of Everything goes to the movies! You will realize the truly universal applicability of the Science not only to your body as a system but also to understand stories and movies as systems.

Onward!

PART 1

The Journey to Systems

CHAPTER 1

A Child of Oppression and Truth

Like most people, when I look back on my life I see things that seem obvious now, but were invisible when they were actually taking place. I see connections that were waiting to be recognized, but I had to learn to see and understand them.

I have a Ph.D. in systems biology from MIT, for example, but long before I studied the science of systems theory, I had already experienced the presence and power of systems throughout my life. Later in this book you'll learn much more about what systems are and what they can do. But for now, I'll just say that I was born into the caste system of India, I was also introduced as a child to the Indian system of medicine and its wisdom tradition known as Siddha, and later I spent a good amount of time in the caste system of American academia, business, and entertainment.

And, in 1978, I built the first email system and later had to endure the rage, collusion, and deplorable vitriol, starting in 2012 after my work was received by the Smithsonian, of those who sought to destroy me for my daring to assert my rightful place in history as the inventor of email. The truth of a 14-year-old, Indian immigrant boy inventing email in Newark, New Jersey was antagonistic to the priesthood of vested interests, "historians," and "internet pioneers" who wished to perpetuate their gated and well-defined caste system of when, where and by whom innovation could take place.

All of this, of course, has made the study of systems a major focus of my life and work -- but if someone were to ask me what conclusions I've come to regarding my experience with systems, I would have to say I have mixed feelings.

I have certainly seen the limiting and destructive effects of the Indian caste system, and also of the surprisingly similar system that exists in America. In fact, I want to do everything I can to reveal those systems for what they are and destroy them if possible. Yes, destroy them. If that sounds like a radical aspiration, that's exactly what I intend.

On the other hand, I have also seen how Siddha --- another system --- a 5,000 year old system of healing and spirituality, had enormous benefits both for both the physical well being and the spiritual health of the community. Watching my grandmother, who was a Siddha healer, was one of the most important experiences of my life. It showed me the practical benefits and spiritual wisdom that could exist in a system that pre-dated Western science by many centuries. It further showed me that none of this depended on the conventional educational system, and definitely not on academic degrees. When I returned to India years later, I also realized how Siddha anticipated many of the elements of modern systems theory. The terminology was different, but the principles were the same.

There will be much more to say about all this throughout the book. But to begin, I was born in Bombay (now called Mumbai), a cosmopolitan and diverse metropolis with the largest population of any city in India. But I also spent large amounts of time in a small village called Muhavur where my grandparents lived. My grandparents were very small family subsistence farmers --- they tilled the Indian soil growing cotton, coconuts, peanuts and rice.

My grandmother worked in the fields for sixteen hours a day. As I've said, she was also a healer in the traditional Indian system of health called Siddha. This is one of the world's oldest healing systems, and it also anticipates and uses the modern systems approach that you'll learn about in a later chapter.

She could predict what was going on in a person's body simply by looking at that person's face. This skill or art is known in the ancient Indian Tamil treatises as *Samudkrika Lakshanam*. After she diagnosed someone, she could provide a healing modality -- it could include massage, or yoga, or a variety of herbs -- always in sync with the person's specific needs and identity. And that, by the way, is the direction that Western science is now trying to take. It's called *personalized medicine* or *precision medicine* --- giving the right treatment, at the right time, for the right person.

My understanding of the knowledge of Siddha and its teachers, known as Siddhars, began by observing my grandmother. Each morning, my grandmother, Chinnathai, would rise before sunrise and, following an ancient tradition, create beautiful drawings known as *kolams* on the ground in front of the entrance to the house. She used milled white rice flour that flowed through her hands, like sand passing through an hourglass, to make abstract geometric and symmetric designs, resembling mandalas.

The kolams served a dual purpose: The rice flour attracted ants and other insects and kept them from entering the home, but there was always a larger, more important, spiritual benefit for the artist and the viewer. Sometimes I would wake up early just to watch my grandmother drawing the daily kolam, a process that was indescribable, with visions emanating from her mind's eye onto the red brown earth. The designs were said to evoke the spiritual world and put one who looked upon them into higher states of consciousness.

Coming home, the kolams were reminders that one was entering a special place. Two solid teak doors were the entrance into a small 10-foot by 12-foot space, which served as the living room, dining room, and the first floor sleeping room. Ahead, one could see the kitchen, where something was always cooking. The fragrance of cumin, ginger, cardamom, red pepper, and freshly ground coconut filled the air. Pictures of the great deities and heroes lined the edge of where the four walls met the ceiling of the living room.

A powerful image of Shiva, my namesake, with the power to destroy, create, and transform; Rama, the virtuous and noble hero of the Ramayana; Devi, the mother Goddess; Parvathi, wife, loyal and devoted consort of Shiva; Ganesha, the elephant headed one who removed obstacles; Jesus, God's avatar and the Savior of mankind; Saraswati, the Goddess of knowledge; Lakshmi, the Goddess of wealth and others. The smell of subtle incense and holy ash was always in the air. My favorite was the deity Muruga, whose picture graced the small altar. Muruga was known as the teacher of teachers or yogi of yogis; the deity's familiar mount was the peacock and above the picture hung a beautiful single peacock feather.

My grandmother knew the ancient arts and was known to be clairvoyant; on occasion she would channel spirits. She had knowledge of the great herbs and medicines to be used for nearly any ailment, and would do rituals and mantras to heal those who requested. Her arms were marked with amazing tattoos. She had a nose ring. Her hair was pitch black and she chewed tobacco and betel leaf. Her face was like the earth, dark with hues of red, and eyes that extended to the beyond, and lines marking her journey across many life times. I thought everyone had a grandmother like her.

She had grown up in Burma, the land of cobras and Buddhism. After giving birth to my father, she did not have another child, something which, at the time, was seen as heresy. There was serious talk of marrying another woman to my grandfather. She and my dad, then five years old, made pilgrimages to many Buddhist temples seeking blessings. One monk with a face my father describes as "pure light," gave my father a mantra, a sacred sound, initiating him to meditation, along with a gold Burmese coin, and a promise that on December 2, he would have a brother. My uncle Siva was born exactly as predicted and to this day wears that Burmese coin as an amulet. My grandmother then went on to have six other children.

My great-grandfather, who I remember well, was also a hardworking farmer and was considered by local villagers also as a Swamiji, a spiritual Master or Adept, who could perform what we in the West would consider superhuman feats. He was her teacher and trained her in many of the ancient arts. My grandmother had a profound understanding of the power of observation and its ability to reveal Nature's hidden secrets. From her, I learned that all things in Nature are interconnected, and that our intentions are the source of our liberation or bondage.

Every day people would come to her house, asking for healing help; on weekends, long lines extended from her door. No one was refused; no payment was ever required. This was not her occupation; her "day job" was working in the rice and cotton fields to make ends meet. My grandmother often talked to me about healing. She said to heal people one had to have the attitude of a warrior with a desire to serve; she said that being able to serve others was a gift from God.

She was the youngest of sixteen children—the only daughter—and the last remaining member of her family; all her siblings had died. She adored her father, who she described as Robin Hood. He literally stole from the rich and gave to the poor, and was beloved by all. She loved to tell me stories of him and the great epics of Indian lore, of Gods and Demons, good and evil, how virtue and honor always overcame deceit and control.

Gossip was never allowed in her home. At night, she would have me lay my head in her lap and tell me those ancient epic stories. I would always ask her what they meant. She would counsel me gently of the age-old truths of being true, kind, courageous and standing up for those who were less fortunate, reminding me that we are Spirit, and the more we were good, the more God's light would shine through our eyes and face.

She would tell me stories about the great Rama, who fought the evil Ravana, who had stolen Sita his beloved wife. Rama was bold and fought with honor, finally overcoming Ravana and bringing back his wife home to safety. That great epic of the *Ramayana*, the valiant journey of Rama, embedded in me a grand and uncompromising idealism for making the world a better place.

Living in Mumbai I was also exposed to the deplorable realities of India's caste system. My earliest memories, as a five-year-old, was realizing that we were "untouchables" --- low castes.

After playing soccer, I remember going to a nearby house with a friend to get some water. I was asked to stand outside, not allowed to enter, and given water in a markedly different kind of cup --- not the normal silverware. I later asked my mom what this meant. She said that we were low castes, and the home was that of an upper caste, and such segregation was how it was in India.

She shared with me how when she went to get water at the village well --- the upper caste would yell out to her as though she was a dirty animal and say, "shoo, shoo Shudra." The word "Shudra" is as derogatory and demeaning as the word "Nigger." She was only allowed to get water when they were not there.

So, as a child I wanted to understand not only the systems of ancient medicine my grandmother practiced to heal others but also the larger systems of oppression such as the caste system, and how to overcome and destroy it to bring truth, freedom and health to the world. Quite an ambition for a young child.

CHAPTER 2

The Invention of Email

It was these multiple worlds of Mumbai and
Muhavur that I was exposed to during my formative
years --- and it was that world I took with me when in
1970 my family emigrated from India to New Jersey, on
my seventh birthday.

My parents made this move for two reasons. First,
we were considered, as I shared, "untouchables" in the
Indian caste system, and, in spite of their incredible
capabilities and achievements as low-caste Indians, they
had hit a ceiling for advancement in India -- and
secondly, they wanted to find better educational
opportunities for their kids --- my sister and me.

However, 1970 was not a good year economically in
America. There was a recession underway and the
original job my father had been offered in Chicago didn't
work out as the recession had caused layoffs and job
reductions. So, we moved first to Paterson, New Jersey,

one of the poorest cities in the country, where my dad found an alternate job.

During my early years in New Jersey, I was certainly encouraged to do well in school, but I was also very much into sports. I wasn't the typical nerd. I was into baseball and soccer -- but I completed all the school's math courses, including Calculus, by the ninth grade, and even published a paper in a mathematics journal as a teenager. I did well in school for a very specific reason. I had been inspired by my grandmother and I wanted to learn medicine and healing. I had very practical goals.

At that time in 1977, the Courant Institute for Mathematical Science at NYU had started a new innovative program in which only forty young students were invited to come to NYU to study an intensive program in Computer Science --- an emerging field as computers themselves were very new.

This program was created by a visionary professor named Henry Mullish. He saw that software programming would one day be a primary need in the high tech revolution that was just beginning, and the United States would need software engineers. I was one of the forty students selected, and I learned eight programming languages at NYU. It was a twelve hour per day program and it went on for over two months. I was the only Indian in the program, and I was also the youngest student. I finished number one in the class.

Getting to NYU from New Jersey involved taking buses and trains, starting at around five in the morning. I'd arrive in New York around seven, and then walk to the University through the colorful and sometimes threatening environment that was New York in those days.

When the NYU program finished, I was very bored by the idea of going back to high school. I was even thinking about dropping out. Fortunately my mom had gotten a degree in statistics in India at a time when it was very unusual, or even revolutionary, for a woman to do anything like that. She was working as a systems analyst at a small, three-campus medical school called the University of Medicine and Dentistry of New Jersey (UMDNJ). Her job was located at the Newark campus of UMDNJ.

My mother introduced me to a scientist named Dr. Swamy Laxminarayan who had a large amount of data on the sudden crib death of infants in their sleep --- also known as SIDS. He asked me to explore the data using artificial intelligence and pattern analysis techniques to see if there was a correlation between infants' sleep patterns and crib death. I developed computer software algorithms to find such correlations. This was my introduction to AI and pattern analysis of what we today call "big data."

The results of my study were later published as a scientific paper at a major medical conference in Finland. This was very exciting and gratifying for me, since it was directly connected to my interest in medicine and healing. I was on my chosen path.

It turned out, however, that my ability to program the computer and work on sleep patterns had attracted the attention of another visionary scientist. His name was Dr. Leslie P. Michelson, and he was a brilliant PhD in experimental particle physics from Brookhaven Labs who was now at UMDNJ. Dr. Michelson had created the Laboratory Computer Network (LCN) which connected the three campuses of Newark, Piscataway and New Brunswick, in New Jersey. This network had nothing to do with the ARPANET or internet, etc. It was an independent network.

Dr. Michelson was also developing new scientific computing software applications to support research at UMDNJ. He had set high standards for any software that was created in his small computer lab at UMDNJ. It had to be bulletproof -- which meant it had to be highly reliable -- and it also had to be user friendly. I was only fourteen years old, but Dr. Michelson didn't treat me like a child. He wanted to challenge me. He wanted to push me as far as I could go.

Dr. Michelson told me about the interoffice mail system that was then used at UMDNJ, and was also used all over the country. He then challenged me to create software that would literally be an electronic replacement for the interoffice paper mail system that connected approximately one thousand offices at the three campuses of UMDNJ. The system I built included an Inbox, Outbox, Drafts, Folders, Memo, Attachments, Carbon Copies (including Blind Carbon Copies), Return Receipt, Address Book, Groups, Forward, Compose, Edit, Reply, Delete, Archive, Sort, and Bulk Distribution. I accomplished this task by writing nearly 50,000 lines of computer code across a system of 35 computer programs which I named "email" -- a term never before

25

used in the English language. It was not a simple system, but a sophisticated enterprise class system.

It worked, was successful, and was used across the university. I wrote a user's manual, held user training sessions and maintained the system by fixing issues and adding new features --- all of this while finishing up some remaining courses in high school.

This whole experience was certainly a major turning point in my life. Creating a major invention like email was of course important. But even at the time I was aware that Dr. Michelson's giving me this assignment represented a complete and total rejection of any caste system -- yes, even in America -- based on age, race, or nationality. He opened the gates for me --- where a 14-year-old boy was invited to work alongside those who were three to five decades older, in a collegial environment, where I was treated no less, with the only expectation being that my work, the product of my labor, would be the judge of my stature --- nothing else.

This was freedom in the interests of science and innovation, and nothing else mattered. I wish I could say that everyone I've encountered in years since then has been as free from prejudice as Leslie Michelson, but that hasn't been the case. As a result, my work has often involved not only a search for innovation, but for justice as well.

At that time, in terms of electronic communication, earlier work had been done on sending rudimentary text messages between computers. But I want to emphasize that email was not just exchanging text messages. Email is a *system* with many interconnected parts that would enable collaboration in the electronic world as the interoffice mail system did in the world of paper and the physical world. Email was a full replica of the secretary's desktop along with all the communication features needed to transact business in an office environment.

Subsequently I won a Westinghouse Science Honors Award for creating email, and I was accepted at MIT. In fact, when I first arrived at MIT, the front page of the MIT newspaper featured three of the 1,041 incoming students' work, and I was one of them for having created email.

Email became something I had done in the past, I didn't focus on it, but I didn't entirely forget about it either. Upon attending MIT, in September of 1981, I learned from the MIT President Dr. Paul E. Gray during dinner at his home that the Supreme Court was not recognizing software patents; however, he advised me to Copyright my invention, since the recent Computer Software Act of 1980 allowed inventors to protect their software inventions using Copyright. That is what I did.

On August 30, 1982, the United States government awarded me the first U.S. Copyright for "Email." I want to emphasize this Copyright was significant since the Supreme Court was not yet recognizing software patents --- a Copyright was the only way to protect software inventions. Therefore, to the greatest extent possible at the time, I was officially recognized as the inventor of email by the United States government.

This sequence of events could have developed very differently if government policies regarding patents had not lagged behind the pace of innovation. Had I been allowed to patent email, I'd now be receiving a penny for every transmission and I'd be a gazillionaire.

CHAPTER 3

Somethings Need to Be Destroyed

Over the next thirty years I sought neither recognition nor financial gain for my invention of email. At MIT I earned four degrees in engineering and design, including a PhD in biological engineering. I was also interested in political systems, since I wanted answers to the oppressive caste system my family and I had experienced in India. I had the opportunity to study with Noam Chomsky, who is both the father of modern linguistics and also one of the most outspoken political thinkers in academia. I learned why and how the Indian caste system came into being --- a historical set of events that very few Indians are even aware of.

During my years at MIT, I always pursued entrepreneurial projects. I was in and out of the university, getting a degree, then leaving to start a company, then getting another degree --- one foot in academia, and one foot out.

By 1993, with the advent of the World Wide Web, email went from being a business application to becoming the dominant form of communication in all fields. At that time, I was doing my PhD in developing a universal AI and pattern analysis system for all sorts of media, including document content, handwriting analysis, and speech signals. During this time, the Clinton White House ran a competition to find an AI solution to their problem of email overload.

The White House had twenty interns sorting 5,000 emails a day into 147 predefined categories including education, healthcare, and many more. Each incoming email would be categorized into one of the categories, and then the sender would receive a form letter associated with a category. It was a very time consuming process. In an attempt to bring this situation under control, the government announced the competition for analyzing and sorting the emails. No such thing had ever been done before, because there had been no need for anything like this.

I entered the competition as the only graduate student. The other entrants were five public and private companies. I won and was selected to provide the service.

Out of that experience I started a company called EchoMail, which helped major corporations process large volumes of email from clients and customers. I thought EchoMail would be a two year project. However, it became a ten year enterprise with 300 employees, and I grew it to $250 million in value. I personally made a lot of money.

In the midst of this, in 2003, my advisor called and urged me come back to MIT to finish my PhD. A major global science initiative, called the Human Genome Project, had just ended which mapped the entire human genome. Despite what the scientists had expected, it turned out that human beings have approximately the same number of genes as an earthworm --- about 20,000. In this atmosphere, the field of *systems biology* was coming into its own, saying we needed to look beyond genes as the "answer to everything." We needed to see the interconnections of molecules across the genome and their communication in cells, just as my grandmother had seen how the facial features of someone connected to their bodily functions.

At this time the National Science Foundation (NSF) had issued what they called the "Grand Challenge," comparable to landing on the moon. The challenge was to mathematically model the whole human cell. I returned to MIT and combined my love of computers with my devotion to medicine and created the technology of CytoSolve in response to the NSF challenge. If Email was the electronic version of the interoffice mail communication system, CytoSolve was the electronic version of the molecular communication system. This could mean the final elimination of animal testing in laboratories.

Based on my work on CytoSolve, MIT awarded me a PhD. In that same year in 2007 I received a Fulbright Fellowship to return to India to study Siddha from a systems biology perspective. The front page of MIT's official newspaper, *MIT Tech Talk*, headlined a feature article: "East meets West: Armed with 4 MIT degrees, Shiva Ayyadurai embarks on new adventure."

This had been my childhood aspiration to understand scientifically how my grandmother was able to heal others using Siddha. My training in systems biology at MIT provided me all the necessary skills.

I discovered that the Siddhars had always been systems thinkers. Unlike conventional Western medicine, they were not reductionist. They didn't look at people and their health in a fragmented way. Their view of health was genuinely holistic.

I discovered a common language, a science, that connected Siddha with modern control systems theory. This was a major breakthrough, and would become the basis of my future teaching and curriculum on Systems Health and "The Science of Everything."

On the night before I was set to leave India to return to the US, following completion of my Fulbright research in 2009, I was called to a meeting with the Director General of the Council of Scientific and Industrial Research (CSIR). CSIR was India's largest scientific enterprise comprised of 37 labs across India and over 4,500 scientists. He invited me to serve as the head of the CSIR's new initiative, "CSIR-TECH," to spin out scientific innovations -- innovations that had just been sitting in the lab -- to the general population of India. The idea was to expedite the transition from the lab bench to the masses.

In this role, I developed a strategic plan for unleashing innovation from those labs by implementing an entrepreneurial program. I visited nearly 1,500 CSIR

Indian scientists all over the country and met people who were absolutely brilliant. Amazing innovations were being developed. But these innovations were being sidetracked by administrators and bureaucrats who were jealous and afraid. There was a high level of corruption.

I wrote an honest report in October of 2009 that exposed the sycophancy, corruption and suppression that was taking place in Indian science. Within hours, I was fired, and was later evicted from my home. Death threats followed, and also threats from the Director General to reporters of major papers: they were not to share the facts. I was forced to flee India on a dramatic journey that included a 32-hour train ride to the Nepal border, plane flight to Kathmandu, and three other airplane flights before I was finally back home in Boston.

Prior to my dismissal, I had been awarded the First Outstanding Scientist/Technologist of Indian Origin by the Prime Minister of India, who serves as the President of CSIR. I had been appointed as Additional Secretary in the Indian government, with the highest Scientist Level H posting. Major newspapers, including *The New York Times*, covered the events of my dismissal, in spite of threats from the Director General of CSIR against NY Times reporters. I was commissioned to write an article for *Nature* by the Nature India editor, which I entitled "Innovation Demands Freedom." Shortly after this article was published, the editor of Nature India was threatened by the then Prime Minister's Office, and the article was removed.

Sometime after I returned to Boston, in late 2011, my mother was dying of pulmonary fibrosis. Much to my surprise, she presented me with a suitcase filled with all the artifacts of my early work on email from 1978 -- my fifty thousand lines of code, everything.

One of my colleagues, a professor at Emerson College reviewed the materials and said, "Shiva, you invented email." As I reviewed the materials, I could, however, only think back to the amazing collegial ecosystem at UMDNJ which allowed a 14-year-old boy to innovate and invent email --- far different than the oppressive and draconian feudal system of CSIR in India, which suppressed innovation.

My friend contacted Doug Aamoth, who was the Technology Editor at *Time Magazine*. Doug reviewed the materials carefully over many weeks and wrote a feature article entitled "The Man Who Invented Email," which informed the general public about email's true origin. In 2012, the Smithsonian Institution's National Museum of American History (NMAH) requested and received the artifacts that documented my work, which really did epitomize the American Dream.

On February 16, 2012, an event was held at the Smithsonian to celebrate the acquisition of all that material. It was after that ceremony that controversy began, which is extensively documented on the Internet. The "controversy" was incited by a group calling itself a "special interest group" body of "computer historians" --- these were industry insiders, loyal to the major defense contractor Raytheon/BBN, who had falsely crowned one of its own employees as the "inventor of email."

After three decades of not promoting my work, these people attacked me as if I were a money-hungry

34

opportunist. The online gossip site Gizmodo called me an "asshole," "a dick," and "a fraud." These inspired threats on other blogs that "the curry-stained Indian should be shot and hanged by his dhothi," and expletives such as "nigger Indian."

Why were there such vicious attacks against me? The reason is simple. The idea that a 14-year-old immigrant Indian boy working in an obscure hospital could invent email disrupted the carefully nurtured storyline that major innovations always had to come from the triangle of big corporations, major universities and the military --- what President Eisenhower and Senator Fulbright had referred to as the "military-industrial-academic" complex.

Specifically, concerning email, those innovations had to come from defense contractors. Therefore those defense contractors should receive whatever huge funding they wanted, because so many wonderful things like email came out of that -- which in actuality had not come from military initiatives.

But the facts on who invented email are black and white. There never was a genuine controversy. The whole media storm was fabricated to continue brainwashing Americans with the idea that innovations come from war, and we as Americans should be happy funding war since we get Tang and Velcro --- which by the way also didn't come from military research either.

The attacks on my reputation were libelous and defamatory. However, I was not able to find an attorney to take on this Goliath of an enemy.

In 2016, after four years of attempting to find an attorney, I signed with Charles Harder, who represented the ex-pro wrestler Hulk Hogan in a highly publicized case against Gawker Media. Charles Harder filed a suit against Gawker Media and I was victorious.

On November 3, 2016 Gawker Media settled with me for $750,000 and removed all three defamatory online articles. This was a big victory for the inventor of email, and more importantly it established the truth that innovation, small or large, can occur anytime, anyplace, by anybody.

Immediately after this victory, the response from the defeated cabal of vested interests was exactly what would be expected: a desire for revenge. This was expressed by frantic blog posts stating that "Shiva Ayyadurai didn't invent email."

Their belief seemed to be that, if they said it loud enough, that untruth would become fact. This is a familiar tactic of those in power: repeat a lie loud and long in order to brainwash the masses.

As this false storyline was being created, the establishment cabal then colluded together to further libel and defame me on the very influential Wikipedia site. Within weeks of my legal victory, the cabal rewrote the opening sentences of my Wikipedia page, -- which would be the first item on a Google search -- stating that the only notable achievement of my life was to have created a controversy by asserting myself as the inventor of email.

But in fact there was no longer any controversy, if there ever had been one. The fact is that I had won and that win would be recognized by a payment of $750,000 from the people who had libeled me in contradiction of the facts.

The defamatory articles were removed because the business folks at Gawker Media and Univision did not want to suffer even greater damage to their wallets. Money, in an odd way, can sometimes motivate justice.

My experiences have brought renewed knowledge of how systems work, and that knowledge will be most powerful weapon to destroy whatever systems oppress the broad mass of humanity. At that same time, that knowledge will provide the insight to create and embrace systems that bring us truth, freedom and health --- as did the Siddha system that my grandmother practiced, without any college degrees.

My core mission, in this book and everywhere else, is to bring you an understanding of systems theory and practice. With that understanding, you will see for yourself that truth is an emergent property arising from the interconnections of the components of any system.

Email, therefore, is not a simple exchange of text messages, but a system which emerges from the interconnection of the many components originally resident in the interoffice mail system. Health emerges from complex, dynamic combinations biological elements -- not from one "magic bullet" drug, or diet, or exercise.

In a similar way, real freedom will not emerge from fighting one aspect of the enemy, whether it's racism, sexism, or classism. Freedom will come from defeating the priesthood system of academia, media, politics, and even entertainment that keeps humanity in bondage through a complex interaction of oppression. The ultimate goal of that system is to dehumanize the many by asserting that only the few are innovative, intelligent, beautiful, and all-knowing.

For the great Siddhars, the revolutionaries, the warriors, the heart of their struggle was against these priesthoods and their caste system. Some things do need to be destroyed --- and that caste system is one such thing.

PART 2

Systems Biology

CHAPTER 4

Revolutionary Road

When I enrolled at MIT as a first year student I was of course very oriented toward science, but I also was more socially engaged than many of my classmates. A pair of photographs from MIT expresses these diverging interests. In one, the school's official student newspaper, *The Tech*, had a front page article featuring achievements of three of the 1,041 incoming students. I was one of the three, and my invention of email was highlighted.

A more dramatic photo in several issues later shows me as a 17-year-old undergraduate burning a South African flag on the steps of the MIT Student Center. I had just led a major protest of several thousand students and workers against MIT's investments in apartheid South Africa. I later challenged the MIT administration to provide proper wages for food service workers and increased student enrollment of women, minorities, and those of lower socio-economic background. On the date of my PhD graduation, as I was receiving my degree, I pulled out a big sign, which said "U.S. Out of Iraq." Half the crowd booed me, and the other half cheered.

I was inspired to act on my own, and to organize the local community against inequities, whether thousands of miles away or right at home. That inspiration was fueled by my personal desire to understand and change *systems* --- systems of oppression like the Indian caste system.

My path as a student at MIT, along with my experiences in India, would be the basis for my future work in the new field of Systems Biology --- as this field provided a much needed opportunity for a systems-based approach to biology.

To get started in understanding Systems Biology, let's look at those two words individually. A system is any set of connecting things, working together with a specific goal or purpose. We are all familiar with mechanical systems: Your car is a system; so is your cell phone. Some systems are relatively simple; others are more complicated, containing within them a variety of still other systems.

The house or apartment in which you live is one example; think about the systems it holds, such as electrical, plumbing, and heating. Look around and what do you see? Do you have a washing machine, a dishwasher, a computer, a CD player, a clock, a pencil sharpener, or iPhone? These are all systems.

What about the word "biology"? Biology is the study of all living things. In modern biology, we study life by conducting simple and complex experiments. In biology, as yet there are no mathematical laws, and there may never be. There are no equations available to predict how tall someone will become under various circumstances based on how much food this person eats or what kind of sports he plays. This is different from physics where observations and many experiments have created mathematical laws that always hold true. Biology, therefore, is fundamentally an experimental science and experiments are the key to the knowledge we have thus far acquired.

Systems Biology is a way of applying the science of systems to the study of life, in all its forms. The mission of systems biology is to give us a new way to grasp the complexity of life. It requires integration of multiple disciplines. In recent years nearly every major university has formed a department called Systems Biology. These are actually interdisciplinary departments bringing together scientists, engineers, and designers across the disciplines of engineering, science and the arts. The complexity of Systems Biology requires this level of cooperative research.

One of the most far-reaching applications of systems biology is Personalized Medicine or Precision Medicine. With my continuing interest in medicine that began with my grandmother, Personalized Medicine was one of the things that attracted me to Systems Biology. Personalized Medicine means that one day you will be able to go to your doctor's office (or possibly simply get on the internet) to access your DNA, which has already been stored in a secure information repository, and submit a sample of that day's blood or saliva. Within moments you will get a read out telling you exactly what to eat for that day and what activities you should do to optimize your day's health.

This is revolutionary change, since most medicine is currently based on a "one size fits all." Pharmaceutical companies spend years finding one drug to cure a particular disease across all people. And the poor results are demonstrating year after year that one drug does not work for everyone. In fact, most drugs work effectively for no more than 10% of the population.

Some patients have an immediate positive response to a drug; others have a variety of side effects. A specific drug may not work for certain people, who are subject to certain conditions. Systems biology hopes to cure this fundamental problem. With a molecular understanding of each one of us as individual and unique beings, it will help deliver the right medicine, at the right time, for the right person.

However, we cannot even think about getting there, until we recognize that *reductionism* is the barrier that needs to be overcome to achieve the grand vision of systems biology.

CHAPTER 5

Beyond Reductionism

Since 1687, when Sir Isaac Newton first published his famous work, *Philosophiae Naturalis Principia,* modern science has been based on a simple and reasonably reliable assumption: If you want to understand anything, you need to take it apart. Many of us remember taking that first biology course in high school or middle school.

We most likely began our study of trees by looking at leaves. This has been the accepted approach to all scientific and mechanical problems: Want to understand a watch, take it apart and examine the pieces. Want to figure out why an engine runs? Examine the pieces. Want to figure out how a human being functions? Look at the parts one at a time. In a Newtonian world, if you understand the parts, you can understand the whole. It's certainly easy to understand why this approach can be so appealing. Some things are simply too complex and huge to grasp any other way. It's complicated so we reduce it down to its parts. This approach is known as *reductionism.*

Reductionism has contributed greatly to human knowledge, but it has its limitations. It's easy to see these limitations in medicine when our bodies are approached as though they are broken up, as it were, into a group of organs and limbs, specialties and sub-specialties. A friend of mine recently visited her internist with a sinus infection. The internist sent her to an ear, nose, throat specialist. The ENT examined her and made some recommendations for medication. My friend complained that a post-nasal drip making its way from the sinuses through her throat and into her lungs was giving her a bad cough. The ENT said he was sorry but the cough involved the lungs, and he didn't treat anything below the neck.

As medical consumers, we know how exasperating this can be. We know that we can't always divide our bodies up into parts. We know that the foot bone is connected to the ankle bone and the ankle bone is connected to the shin bone and the shin bone is connected to the knee bone. Yet, if we have a foot pain and a knee pain, we have to visit at least two different doctors, who in all probability are not consulting with each other to determine if there is a connection. This is one of the problems associated with a reductionist approach to health.

Modern science is beginning to realize that a reductionist approach gives only part of the entire picture—only a portion of the truth. When you connect a bunch of things, whether they are auto parts or human parts, something emerges that is greater and different than the sum of its parts. Take something as basic as a clock. If you take a clock apart, it's nothing more than a collection of odd assorted pieces. When it's put together in the right order, with the right connections, a clock assumes an almost magical function in terms of what it does and how a reliance on an accurate reading of time impacts your world. If this is true for a clock, imagine what happens when you are talking about a living organism, whether it is a tree, an animal, or a human being.

Systems theory is a direct pushback against reductionism, particularly with regard to health and wellness. Proponents of systems theory quote Aristotle who clearly stated, "The whole is different from the sum of its parts." A systems approach to health takes the human spirit as well as the mind-body connection into account. Men and women who want to take a more holistic approach to health frequently engage in practices like meditation and yoga; they are more careful about what they eat and look for ways to encourage spiritual as well as physical healing. Modern New Age movements have popularized holistic health practices. And to the shock and often annoyance of some of the medical establishment, these methods sometimes work.

Those who like to point out the failures of so-called "alternative" techniques tend to focus on the word "sometimes." This is a valid criticism. Practitioners of holistic healing can't always satisfactorily duplicate their results. They can't explain successes using the rigors of modern science, which requires standardization and reproducibility; when something works, they can't explain why. Instead of scientific explanations, what we see and hear is a fair amount of hand waving and conversations using buzzwords like "meridians," "detox," and "energy." New Age healing extremists often go too far and throw science completely out the window. This approach encourages people to avoid modern medicine altogether and rely instead on peculiar diets, questionable herbal methods, and unreliable faith healers.

Here's the problem: when the complex system that is your body has a complex illness, a reductionist approach may not give you the healing you need; similarly a new holistic diet combined with meditation or any other alternative method will have its own limitations.

Complex problems require solutions that speak to the big picture, which is where a systems approach is most helpful. A systems-based approach to life may help us find the middle way between reductionism and holism. It helps us understand the whole as an interconnection of parts, not just the sum of its parts. It helps us recognize the values as well as the weaknesses in a Newtonian world model, which implies that there is always a certain linear cause and effect predictability.

CHAPTER 6

Systems of Systems

A systems-based approach to biology emerges where reductionism ends. Reductionist thinking and the central dogma of Watson and Crick had emphasized that genes alone make us who we are. However, this has proven to be completely wrong.

Since biology is the primary source of knowledge and insight for developing healthcare treatments, the necessary and significant changes to advance modern healthcare, therefore, cannot take place without changes in how biology itself is practiced. Biology today, unlike physics or engineering, is based on experiments rather than first principles, *ab initio*. Biologists do many experiments to understand genes, proteins, and protein-protein interactions.

The all-time largest and most ambitious experiment in biology was the Human Genome Project (HGP,) begun in 1990 and completed around 2003.

The HGP was predicated on the hypothesis that what made a human different from a nematode, a worm, was the number of genes. Originally, it was estimated that a human had approximately 100,000 genes. But the HGP concluded that humans have only 20,000 to 25,000 genes, far less than what was originally theorized. This was almost the same number of genes as the 19,000 genes possessed by the nematode *Caenorhabditis elegans*. The genome of the starlet sea anemone *Nematostella vectensis*, a delicate animal only a few inches long, has approximately 18,000 genes.

Regardless of whether human or nematodes or sea anemone have similar numbers of genes, the HGP revealed great differences in their complexity of function as whole organisms. This apparent contradiction led biologists to conclude that perhaps the number of genes in the genome is not directly connected an organism's complexity. Instead, much of that complexity can be ascribed to regulation of existing genes by other substances (such as proteins) rather than to novel genes. Molecular interactions across the nucleus, cytoplasm, and organelles -- beyond the number of genes in the nucleus itself -- may be a critical element in determining the difference between a human and a worm.

This reasoning has led to an even greater determination to understand the structure of proteins (e.g. the product of genes) and protein–protein interactions. In short, the HGP demonstrated that we are not our genes --- that who we are is likely something that emerges from the complex interplay of genes and the products of genes interacting in ways where genes can be turned on and off.

These results mean that we need to move to *systems* biology that focuses attention not only on the genome, but on the complex interaction of "systems of systems" across genes, proteins, and molecular pathways. All these are influenced by an "epigenetic" layer affected by both endogenous and exogenous systems including nutrition, environment, and perhaps even thoughts that affect genes themselves.

This system of systems approach aims to create a holistic model of the whole organism by integrating the complexity of systems of systems from molecule, to molecular pathways, to large-scale organization, as illustrated below:

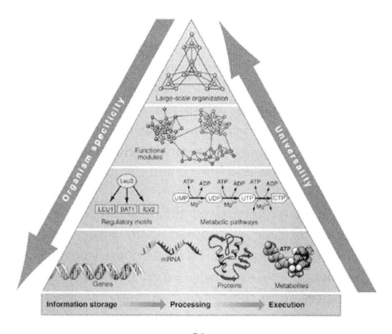

An important attribute of the complexity pyramid is the gradual transition from the particular (at the bottom level) to the universal (at the top.) Integrated models can represent the most compact, unambiguous, and unified form of biological hypotheses, and as such they could be used to quantitatively explore interrelationships at both the molecular and cellular levels.

Although systems biology is a new field, building a systems-level understanding of biology is not a new phenomenon. More than 5,000 years ago, traditional systems of medicine including Siddha, Unani, Ayurveda, and Traditional Chinese Medicine (TCM) proposed systems approaches to describe the whole human physiome. In modern times, starting in 1930s with the concept of homeostasis and biological cybernetics, attempts were made to understand biology at a systems level using the languages of physics and control systems engineering.

Systems biology is now developing a systems-level understanding by connecting our knowledge of activity at the molecular level to higher-level biological functions. Previous attempts at system-level approaches were primarily limited to description and analysis of biological systems at the physiological level. Since these approaches had little understanding of how molecular interactions were linked to biological functions, a systems-based biology that connected molecular interactions to biological functions was not possible.

Contemporary systems biology, however, offers a new opportunity to link the behaviors of molecules to the characteristics of biological systems. This new field will enable us to describe the systems of systems of cells, tissues, organs, and human beings within a consistent framework governed by the basic principles of physics.

CHAPTER 7

Modeling the Whole Cell

In 2003, after having been the CEO of EchoMail, Inc. for nearly 10 years, my advisor Prof. C. Forbes Dewey asked me to come back to MIT to complete my Ph.D. At that time, as I shared earlier, the Human Genome Project had just ended with the ironic conclusion that humans have about 20,000 genes --- the same number as an earthworm. Not only did this discovery lead to the field of systems biology but also to another development.

This development was the impetus to mathematically model the whole cell. The National Science Foundation (NSF) had put forward this "Grand Challenge" to inspire scientists to create a computer model of the cell. This challenge intrigued me as it provided a unique opportunity to express my love of computing and medicine.

The systems approach here was to consider the cell as a system of interconnected molecular pathways, which were the elemental modules of complex cellular functions. Biological systems were thought to have large number of parts which are related in complex ways. Functionality, therefore, emerges as the result of molecular interactions between many proteins relating to each other in multiple cascades and in interaction with the cellular environment.

Computing these molecular interactions could determine the logic of healthy and diseased states. One way to model the whole cell would be through a "bottom up" reconstruction of the human metabolic network, which was done primarily through a manual process of integrating databases and pathway models.

It was possible to regard molecular networks as systems that decode and transform complex inputs in time, space, and chemistry into combinatorial output patterns of signaling activity. In this way, accurate experimentation and detailed modeling of network behavior in terms of molecular properties could reinforce each other. The goal then becomes a linking of molecular pathway models on small parts to build larger models in order to form detailed kinetic models of larger chunks of molecular pathways, such as metabolism, for example, and ultimately of the entire living cell.

Integrating systems of molecular pathways demonstrates how integrated networks show emergent properties that the individual pathways do not possess -- including extended signal duration, activation of feedback loops, thresholds for biological effects, or a multitude of signal outputs. In this sense, a cell can be seen as an adaptive autonomous agent or as a society of such agents, where each can exhibit a particular behavior depending on its cognitive capabilities.

Unique mathematical frameworks would be needed to obtain an integrated perspective on these complex systems, which operate over wide length and time scales. These may involve multi-layered, hierarchical approaches, in which the overall signaling network at one layer is modeled in terms of effective "circuit" or "algorithm" modules. Then, at other layers, each module is correspondingly modeled with more detailed incorporation of its actual underlying biochemical and biophysical molecular interactions.

The mammalian cell may be considered as a central signaling network connected to various cellular machines that are responsible for phenotypic functions. Cellular machines such as transcriptional, translational, motility, and secretory machinery can be represented as sets of interacting components that form functional local networks.

As biology began to move into the post-genomic era, a key emerging question concerns the understanding of complex molecular pathways functioning as dynamical systems. Prominent examples include multi-molecular protein "machines," intracellular signal transduction cascades, and cell–cell communication mechanisms. As the proportion of identified systems involved in any of these molecular pathways continues to increase, the daunting challenge of developing useful models – both mathematical and conceptual - for how they work was drawing increased interest.

Multi-scale modeling, I realized, would be essential to integrating knowledge of human physiology -- starting with genomics, molecular biology, and the environment through the levels of cells, tissues, and organs -- all the way to integrated systems behavior. The lowest levels concern biophysical and biochemical events. The higher levels of organization in tissues, organs, and organism are complex, representing the dynamically varying behavior of billions of cells interacting together.

Biological pathways can be seen to share structural principles with engineered networks, along with three of the most important shared principles: modularity, robustness to component tolerances, and use of recurring circuit elements.

These insights led me, as a part of my MIT Ph.D. research, to create CytoSolve --- "Cyto" meaning cell and "Solve" meaning solving. CytoSolve was created to be new computer-based platform for integrating systems of biological pathway models. I also refer to it as a "collaboratory" --- meaning the different engineering components of the cell could be organized, modeled and then integrated together through collaboration.

CytoSolve is a system that enables computational collaboration and integration --- not that different than email. If email is the system that was the electronic replica of the mail communication system, then CytoSolve is the electronic replica of the molecular communication system. More importantly, just as email was a revolution in communication, CytoSolve is a revolution in medicine.

Within 11 months, for example, CytoSolve was used to discover a combination therapy of drugs that was shown to perform *in silico* (on the computer) better than the current "gold standard" for pancreatic cancer. Our combination received FDA allowance to proceed to clinical trials within that 11 months. The possibilities of CytoSolve's applications for medicine and health are limitless.

PART 3

The First Systems Biology

CHAPTER 8

Siddha and Ayurveda

After completing my Ph.D. in systems biology in 2007, I wanted to take some time off from academia to go back to the field and pursue my childhood dream to understand how my grandmother was able to heal those villagers. How did Siddha, that ancient system of Indian medicine, work? I felt that my training at MIT provided me a solid foundation in both Western biology as well as in engineering. This foundation could be used to apply a rigorous scientific and critical approach in understanding Siddha. Funding from the Fulbright Fellowship provided me the opportunity to pursue this research, entitled "Siddha to Systems Biology."

A detailed review of Siddha (and Ayurveda as it is known in Northern parts of India) will provide a framework for you to appreciate the journey to the Science of Everything. Siddha and Ayurveda are ancient systems of Indian medicine that have been practiced for over 5,000 years.

Siddha is from the Tamil word meaning "perfection." Ayurveda means "knowledge of life," from the words "ayus" (life) and "veda" (knowledge.) Siddha is predominantly practiced in southern India, while Ayurveda is mainly practiced in the north. Siddha and Ayurveda have particular differences, such as emphasis on particular modalities and minor variations in terminology, but their foundational elements are the same.

We in the West tend to think that the scientific system that has been built here is the only legitimate one. This is not true. Scientific methods have been used for thousands of years in places Westerners do not normally think of as having anything in common with American or European colleges and universities.

When I came to MIT as a first year student, I remember walking onto 77 Massachusetts Avenue and standing on the steps of the domed building; I immediately noticed how much it resembled the temples I knew in India. Thousands of years ago, before what we now call the Common Era, Siddha teachers, who occupied those temples and used nature as their laboratory, developed disciplined scientific methods and approaches.

These Siddhars, or "Rishis," were scientists, no different than a modern research scholar or professor. They conducted detailed research, experimented, taught, took on students and published through song and poetry. They developed an understanding of nature that recognized the individuality of each of human being, and found ways to link that individuality to the interconnected system of nature around them. They solved problems that we are only now beginning to investigate, so it behooves us to take them seriously.

As I've mentioned earlier, my interest in medicine and my knowledge of the Siddhars began by observing my grandmother, Chinnathai. One truth that my grandmother shared with me, at an early age, was The Law of Karma: "For every cause there is an effect." When my grandmother said these words, she was reminding me that everything in life is interconnected. Drop a pebble into a stream, and it sets off a series of consequences; ripples have meaning.

Ancient sages also referenced these words, which for millennia were seen as merely a poetic or spiritual statement of the concept of Karma, and, unfortunately, sometimes used to rationalize oppression and one's lot in life. However when Isaac Newton echoed a similar allegory, "For every action there is an equal and opposite reaction" and demonstrated the reality of these words through modern science, the words took on a material reality, beyond religious obfuscations, and changed the course of modern history.

Newton demonstrated how physical bodies interact and predicted the motion of these interactions with precision. His discovery, known as Newton's Law of Motion, unleashed the creation of modern science and society. The reality he unraveled created modern machines, bridges, airplanes, cars, skyscrapers, and spaceships that landed on the moon. Newton's insights and experiments gave concrete meaning to the spiritual concept of Karma.

I learned about Karma as a child in India. Here in America, when I learned about Newton's Law of Motion, I couldn't help but relate it back to my grandmother's words. It seemed fairly apparent to me that Newton and the Indian sages my grandmother so often referenced were saying the same thing. Both Newton and the Siddhars were wise men who came to their conclusions using their powers of observation. Newton arrived at his conclusions through the power of observation, which he wrote down as math equations.

But there was no available mathematical language for Newton to use so he developed his own—calculus. When we think of the original Siddha elders, we don't think of them as scientists. Yet, they were. Like Newton, they were using the oldest scientific methods of observation; their university was all of nature. Siddha practitioners observed the body. They watched breath, listened to heartbeats, recognized the importance of thoughts and intentions. Their wisdom is all arrived at through observation.

I was constantly amazed by what my grandmother knew just from looking at a person's face. Her powers of observation, without the help of any instruments, were incredible. She saw colorings, marks, moles, lines, locations and asymmetries. Her mind and training connected these features to areas of imbalance in the body.

After determining the issues, she would then prescribe a treatment. Sometimes, she suggested the taking of an appropriate herb; other times she prescribed the repetition of certain sounds or mantras; when necessary, she performed a body manipulation. These treatments were aimed at correcting the imbalances she diagnosed from the face. It sounds amazing, but my grandmother was able to diagnose someone's problem simply by observing his or her face. She was able to prescribe treatments that worked.

My grandmother's skills at face reading and her medical treatments were based on Siddha methods and teachings. The 5,000 year old Siddha medical system is one of the oldest in the world, and the oldest still practiced. Siddha medicine is an Indian system developed in the Southern Indian region of Tamil. The word Siddha means "fully perfected" or "enlightened." Most of us have heard the name "Siddhartha" or "enlightened one" used in reference to the Buddha who lived some 2,500 years ago.

The ancient teachings say the Siddha system was directly transmitted by Lord Shiva to his wife Parvathi. Parvathi then gave the knowledge to one of her two sons, Muruga. Muruga, a Hindu deity, then transmitted it to Agastya, a sage, who is known as the father of Siddha medicine. Agastya, in turn, passed these teachings and knowledge on to seventeen other Siddhars.

These eighteen highly evolved beings, regarded as spiritual saints, then established a lineage of information and wisdom that has come down to us over the centuries. The Siddha scriptures are practical as well as esoteric and contain teachings on all aspects of life including science, meditation, yogi, alchemy, tantra, medicine, art, enlightenment, and herbal treatments.

People often wonder how all this could have been transmitted in such complete form for so many years. In ancient India, the Siddha scriptures were preserved by scribes who carefully etched Siddha wisdom, including medical formularies, onto treated palm leaves. The etched lettering was then treated with dyes made from coal black or turmeric. These palm leaves formed collections of manuscripts that could last for centuries. When these treasured manuscripts started to deteriorate, new scribes went to work, using the same methods. Thousands and thousands of palm leaf manuscripts have been passed down in this way. Currently, scholars and specialists have started work collecting, transcribing, and cataloguing what has been found.

Many of the texts saved in this way focus on the use of herbal medicinal formularies, face reading, sound, crystals, as well as different types of yoga, visualization, and meditation. There were even texts devoted to art and drawing—what we would now call art therapy. In India, the Siddha medical system continues to be practiced today, and you can still get a Siddha MD degree. Siddhars are also renowned as artists and poets, and much of the teachings handed down through time are in the form of songs and poetry. It's interesting to note that in these ancient teachings, medicine is viewed as both science and art.

CHAPTER 9

Layers of Meaning

The texts of Siddha were written in poetic form which could be recited as a poem or a song. Each poem had two meanings. There was the apparent or face value meaning of the poem, and then there was the medical or more esoteric meaning, which revealed a higher truth.

The apparent meaning enabled lay people to enjoy the poem as a work of art. The more esoteric meaning could only be deciphered by those who were either their disciples or had the acumen and intuition to see beyond the visible meaning. In some sense, the Siddhars presented even their knowledge in visible and invisible forms, requiring one to perceive the invisible and understand it, to reveal the real meaning and truth behind the verse.

Consider the following example of a simple poem, which is written in Tamil as follows:

Mangai paal vundu
Malaimai irruporkuu

Thengai paal
Eythikkadi kuthambai

Here's an English translation:
  Those drinking mango milk
  And living on a hill
  Coconut milk,
  Is not needed

At face value, this poem relates the power of mango milk. For anyone who has seen a mango on a tree, will notice a small amount of white milk, like sap, comes from the stem when the mango is plucked. This milk is normally ignored and seen as nothing significant having no value. The poem states that this seemingly insignificant milk has a powerful nutritional value to those living on a hill; and this value, is even more potent than the highly nutritious and valued coconut milk.

But a Siddhar disciple would, however, decipher the poem, beyond that apparent and literal meaning, as follows: The hill represents the top of the head --- the "hill" of the human body. The mango is the pineal gland, located between the two eyebrows on top of the head. The mango milk is the hormone, melatonin, however small the amount, the pineal gland secretes through the right meditative practices. According to the Siddhars, this "milk" is an elixir, far healthier than any food in the world, including coconut milk, which the Siddhars considered one of the most nutritious foods.

Siddhars codified their knowledge in poetic verses with dual meanings to ensure that the truths were made accessible to those who had the right training. They recognized the immense power of their teachings, acquired over many millennia of scientific observation and experimentation, and wanted to protect them from those who could misuse it or did not have the relevant training to use it appropriately. Over the many centuries, Siddhars have continued to take this approach, passing it on to only their most trusted followers.

The Indo-Aryan invasions resulted in much of the Siddhars' knowledge being suppressed; some of it was incorporated into Vedic texts, such as Ayurveda, which many in the West are more aware of. Furthermore, the British invasion resulted in the suppression of many of the Indian traditional practices in favor of western medicine. Today, unlike my grandmother, the average Indian interested in medicine are taught that traditional systems of medicine such as Siddha are inferior to Western medicine.

Fortunately in 2005 after much lobbying by those who were interested in bringing Siddha to the modern world, the government of India inaugurated the National Institute of Siddha, in the southern state of Tamil Nadu. This Institute today is focused on converting the hundreds of thousands of the ancient Siddha texts written in Tamil poetry. Over the next few years, more and more knowledge of the Siddhars art and medicine will be made available.

Hundreds of thousands of palm leaves are filled with this kind of artistic poetry which reveal both an apparent concept and a more hidden and valuable truth. The original teachings of Siddha stressed enlightenment or spiritual perfection, but it's important to note that Siddhars taught that enlightenment and physical health are intrinsically linked. They believed that methods that strengthened one's physical well being would lead to greater spiritual growth. To this end, they developed practices emphasizing diet, yoga, and meditation that would help practitioners become healthier as they sought to become Siddhars or "perfected ones."

My grandmother told me that Siddhars believed that the entire cosmos, from the smallest particle to the largest solar systems, were connected by consciousness and energy. Siddha practitioners taught, "As above, so below." If you want to understand natural law, start by observing the dynamics of your own body. Understand yourself, and you will understand the whole world.

Over thousands of years, the Siddhars developed and organized a holistic system of understanding based on observable patterns of interaction. Here in the West, Systems biology is building an understanding of the universe bottom-up from cell to tissue to organs to intact organism.

Siddha, on the other hand, understands the world top-down as energy permeating from the cosmos to the ecosystem, to human, to organs to tissue. As I continued my study of Siddha medicine and Systems Biology, I came to recognize the potential of integrating Siddha and Systems Biology to build a convergent understanding of life, integrating the top-down and bottom up approaches of ancient and modern medicine.

CHAPTER 10

Siddha's Model of a Human Being

The Siddhars taught that there is a temple within each of us. But what exactly does that mean? Is this a spiritual concept? And where exactly is this temple located? How do we find it?

The concept of a "temple within" is <u>not based</u> on mysticism. The ancient Siddhars were considered radicals because they opposed many of the mystical religious traditions then prevalent in India. They were focused on the quest for Truth and that state of perfection, known as Siddhi. They were against codified scriptures, superstition, blind devotion, and guru worship. Although they were not atheistic or agnostic, they had no real concept of deities as we think of them now. They considered themselves scientists, not mystics.

In the Siddha tradition, everything is related to science: it all started with unmanifest energy, which they called Purusha or consciousness. When consciousness awakens, energy appears and interacts; and then Nature unfolds from energy to matter, through various levels. Siddha is about understanding not only the body but also the nature of all things that interact with the body including the larger systems from the microscopic to the macroscopic. But Siddha concepts concerning the human body and the physical nature of man are quite different from what we learn here in the West.

The Siddhars as scientists developed their precise model of a person based on their experiments and observations. They came to the fundamental conclusion that the human body possessed a complete infrastructure to find truth at all levels of existence.

This thesis is different from the Western view of the human being. Siddha research led to an important conclusion, one as real as gravity: each one of us is made up of three separate and interconnected systems: The Visible Body; The Invisible Body; and the Atman, the infinite and unknowable.

Western medicine is primarily concerned with the physical or visible body. Siddhars said that if we want to understand the puzzle that is man, we need to take all three systems into account. If we fail to do this, we are not seeing the whole picture.

An important point to remember: Siddhars taught that both the visible self and the invisible self were part of the manifest material world. In short, both the seen and the unseen human systems are described as a continuum between matter and energy --- the visible self having more matter and the invisible self being composed of more energy. They acknowledged that some things are not visible to the human eye but that doesn't make them any less real and tangible. Here, again, are the three systems that make up the individual man or woman.

The Visible Self -- Discussions of the Visible Self include all the parts of self that can be heard, felt, smelled, seen or touched.

The Invisible Self -- Discussions of the invisible self include our emotional and spiritual selves; they include our five senses, as well as our various states of mind, including the conscious state, subconscious state, unconscious state, and dream state. Our invisible self also includes our memories, thoughts, wisdom, and common sense, which is called Buddhi (and pronounced boodhi). When I was growing up and my mother wanted to remind me to pay attention to what I was doing, she would tell me, "Use your Buddhi".

The Atman, or soul -- The Siddhas spent very little time discussing the atman or soul and left this in the realm of the unknowable, which could only be experienced by traversing across the visible and invisible worlds within. They focused, instead, on the visible and the invisible self, performing research and study to discover a system to enable each individual to uniquely pursue that journey within, through the right amount of food to support the physical body, and exercises and meditative practices to support the invisible bodies.

CHAPTER 11

The Architecture of Existence

The foundational elements of Siddha and Ayurveda are conveyed in a native systems architecture that organizes and describes all existence, from the smallest and most subtle elements to the largest. This system also reveals core principles that provide a model for regulating one's life towards optimal health.

The systems architecture of Siddha and Ayurveda are presented in a multi-layered fashion with a particular terminology that describes the elements at each layer. To anyone unfamiliar with Siddha and Ayurveda, this terminology may seem obscure or even "mystical." Our immediate focus, therefore, will be to present and explain this terminology layer by layer.

The first layer is known as *Purusha*. Purusha is best described as consciousness, which expresses itself as will, desire, or motivation.

Purusha is said to give rise to *Prakriti*, the second layer, which represents all material existence that is manifested out of Purusha. A goal or an idea, for example, is representative of Purusha. The expression of that idea in some material form is known as Prakriti. In Indian metaphysics, the entire universe was formed from an idea/thought/will/desire (Purusha) that gave rise to the material existence (Prakriti) that we experiences as matter, energy and information.

Prakriti manifests itself in three forms or aspects of energy. These are known as the Gunas: Sattvic, Rajasic, and Tamasic. The Gunas are the "flavors" of Prakriti, each having its own particular subtle qualities. The Gunas are qualities of subtle energy that cannot be seen, touched, tasted, heard or smelled.

In the next layer of architecture, however, the Gunas manifest in material forms that can be engaged by the five senses. When the Gunas materialize in this way, they are known as the Panchabuthas, or the "five elements." Unlike modern physics, the term "elements" does not refer to elements from the periodic table, but is closer to "states of matter."

The five elements in the Siddha and Ayurveda terminologies, along with their English translations, are below:

Siddha	Ayurveda	English
Akayam	Akasha	Space
Vayu	Vayu	Air
Thee	Agni	Fire
Neer	Jala	Water
Mann	Prithvi	Earth

Practitioners of Siddha and Ayurveda use the interaction of these five elements to understand the dynamics of all nature. In the human body, the Panchabuthas mix with each other in various proportions to form physiological entities such as tissues, as well as to define the whole organism. The Panchabuthas are important in Indian medicine because they give rise to individual constitutions and body types.

The notion of body constitution is presented in the fifth layer through the concept of three *doshas*. Our bodies are space, in which air circulates; they have "fire," expressed as heat; and they have solid structure, made of water and earth. Each of these three components is identified with one of the doshas, which are known as *Vata, Pitta* and *Kapha*.

Three Doshas	Panchabuthas
Vata	Space + Air
Pitta	Fire
Kapha	Water + Earth

Every human body is composed of combinations of these elements, and this combination is central to Siddha and Ayurveda's conception of health and well-being. The specific combination of doshas is present at birth and determines the body type of the individual. This body type is known as the individual's *Prakriti*.

The sixth layer is composed of seven *Dhatus*. The Vata, Pitta, and Kapha constituents of an individual control the nature of that person's Dhatus, which are closely related to tissues in human physiology. The

Dhatus, in the Siddha and Ayurveda terminologies, along with their English translation, are in the chart below:

Siddha	Ayurveda	English
Enbu	Asthi	Bone
Cheneer	Rakta	Blood
Moolai	Majja	Marrow
Sukila/Sronitha	Shukra	Reproductive Tissues
Saram	Rasa	Plasma
Oon	Mamsa	Muscle
Kozhuppu	Meddha	Fat

The seventh layer is the *Kosha*, which is the whole body of the organism. The body includes the *Indriyas*, which are the five senses; *Manas,* which represent the mind; and, the *Karmendriyas,* which represent the physical organs.

CHAPTER 12

Vata, Pitta, Kapha

Siddha and Ayurveda are history's first systems biology, as they provide a multi-layered system to understand all life. The terminology may be foreign, but the organization of Siddha and Ayurveda provides a holistic model describing the whole spectrum of existence, from the metaphysical to the intact living organism.

In the language of Siddha and Ayurveda, the three forces of Vata, Pitta and Kapha, in varying levels, define the state of the Dhatus and the Kosha.

Vata is made up of space and air. Vata control the forces of movement, such as motion of the body, or the flow of receiving and sharing information.

Pitta controls the forces of transformation. This includes digestion, for example, or the conversion of an idea into an action.

Kapha controls the forces that provide storage, structure, or containment. The skeleton of the body, the body's storage of fat, and even memory are controlled by Kapha.

The chart below illustrates the systems biology of Siddha and Ayurveda and their foundational elements:

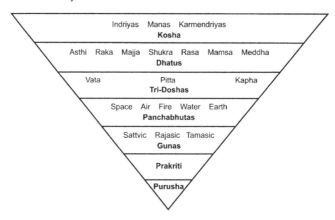

When Siddha medical practitioners look at an individual, they always start with a basic question: "What is this person's basic nature, or Prakriti?" They use a personalized approach to perform diagnostics to get a sense of someone's constitutional makeup, based on his or her combination of *doshas*.

The chart that follows in the next page illustrates the Kosha (the human body), within the large rectangle. The body is defined by the interaction of Vata, Pitta, and Kapha elements. Siddha and Ayurveda recognize that *Karma* (action) leads to *Karma-Phal,* or the "fruits of Karma".

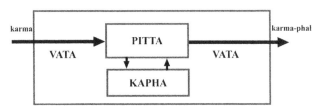

Karma affects Prakriti. For example, the Karma of eating the wrong food or not sleeping enough will lead to Karma-Phal, such as poor skin and being overweight. The Karma-Phal is a symptom of the displacement of the individual's Prakriti. This displaced Prakriti is called *Vikriti*.

Someone's Prakriti may be 30% Vata, 20% Pitta, and 50% Kapha. But due to certain Karmic effects, their Vikriti may become 30% Vata, 50% Pitta, and 20% Kapha. Karma displaced their Prakriti by increasing Pitta and lowering Kapha.

In Siddha and Ayurveda, "health" means an individual's capacity to maintain the body's particular constitution -- Prakriti -- in the midst of stresses and disturbances, through a continuous self-regulating feedback process. This regulatory process is illustrated below:

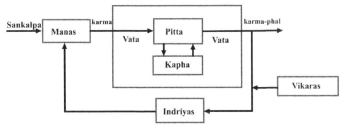

This process begins with a *Sankalpa*, a resolution, to set a goal for optimal health. Optimal health means ensuring that the Kosha (the body) maintains its unique

79

Prakriti, in the midst of *Vikaras* (or disturbances) to the Kosha. Some of these *Vikaras* may be beyond the control of the individual, such as weather changes or moving to a new location. In Siddha and Ayurveda, there is an extensive classification of the different types of Vikaras.

The Manas, the mind, is critical in making the intelligent decisions to input the correct Karma, into the Kosha, which is denoted by the large rectangle in the illustration. The Kosha contains the constitutive elements of Vata, Pitta and Kapha. Based on the Karma, sent into the Kosha, the Vata, Pitta and Kapha elements are adjusted to output Karma-Phal.

The Manas require the *Indriyas* (senses) of smell, taste, hearing, seeing and touch, to be aware of the current Karma-Phal and the Vikaras. Based on the difference between Sankalpa and the Karma-Phal, the Manas make changes to their Karma to adjust the Kosha, to move it away from a state of Vikriti and back to its Prakriti.

The Manas can send certain Karma into the Kosha by varying the intake of certain food, going for a jog, or meditating. This affects the Vata, Pitta, Kapha elements of the Kosha, which results in different Karma-Phal. The process is a constant feedback process, where the Indriyas continually monitor the Karma-Phal and the Vikaras to make adjustments to their Karma, to achieve their Sankalpa.

In summary, there are nine important elements which reflect the core principles of Siddha and

Ayurveda. These nine elements are shown in the chart below:

Element
Karmas
Karma-Phal
Vata
Pitta
Kapha
Sankalpa
Manas
Indriyas
Vikaras

PART 4

Systems Theory

CHAPTER 13

The Systems Toolbox

Perhaps the most important knowledge I got from MIT was modern control systems engineering and systems theory. I'm now going to now share this incredible knowledge with you in two important ways. First, you won't need to go to MIT to get it. Second, I've developed some important new aspects so as to unify and clarify principles to make it far more accessible and understandable for everyone.

Systems theory is a toolbox of practical concepts, similar to the scientific understanding of gravity or electromagnetism. It's a very organized and logical way of comprehending the forces that operate in the world. Using systems theory, things that previously seemed random or mysterious can be understood completely and intelligently.

A system is a set of objects or energies working together for a specific goal or purpose. The first step toward understanding systems theory is recognizing the connections between elements that might once have seemed separate but are actually linked together in a system.

Systems can be simple or infinitely complex. A wristwatch, a cow, a human heart, a city, and a washing machine are all systems – as is the Earth itself and even the whole universe. Your body is a system with many subsystems within it. Once you understand how systems work, you can understand how anything works.

To achieve any goal, you will need to understand how *intelligent systems* function. But before we go there, we will begin by understanding how *open systems* work. A toaster and an electric heater are examples of open systems. But the presence of a self-correcting thermostat makes your home heating system an intelligent system.

All systems include five basic elements: *Input, Output, Transport, Conversion,* and *Structure.*

Input is the stuff coming into a system. There can be a single input or multiple inputs. An input can be information, matter, or energy. For example, what did you have to eat today? Did you get any exercise, or did you stay in bed all afternoon? What did you see out the window? What music did you listen to? Whom did you speak with on the phone?

Output is the stuff coming out of a system. This can be a single output or multiple outputs and, like input, output can be information, matter, or energy. The output is the direct result of the inputs (the karma) into a system. If you somehow plugged your toaster into a nuclear power plant, there would be too much electrical input. This would cause a negative output: your toaster blows up. But if you try to light a city with flashlight batteries, you'll get a negative output for the opposite reason: too little input. Depending on the situation, not enough can be as bad as too much.

Transport is the principle of *movement* in a system: the process of information, matter, or energy moving from input to output, from karma to *karma-phal*, from cause to effect. It's the presence or absence of dynamic progress of stuff moving from source to destination. In a computer, transport is the aspect of the machine's process of moving information, bits of ones and zeroes, through the system, from the keyboard (input) to the screen display (output). When purchasing a computer, you may want one that does this very quickly, or you may need to focus on something else.

Conversion in systems theory refers to the process of transforming or *converting* an Input into an Output. The force of conversion changes information, matter, or energy from one form to another. The Central Processing Unit (CPU) of a computer, along with the necessary software, embodies conversion. When you input three symbols on the keyboard ("1 + 1", for example) the CPU converts those symbols into an output, which is "2."

Structure refers to the boundaries, connections, and overall internal environment <u>within</u> which the activities of transport and conversion take place. Structure is sometimes referred to as the storage aspect of a system. A car, whether it's a racer or a SUV, needs a body or frame made of metal, rubber, and plastic. Both a fighter jet and a passenger plane need the fuselage, which holds the cockpit, seats, and engines. Health, physical strength, and emotional stability are structural aspects of a human system.

CHAPTER 14

Open Systems

An *open system* provides a particular Output from a particular Input. Once the Input is set, the Output is set. A basic electric room heater is another everyday example of an open system.

Assuming the heater is plugged into the wall, turning the heater ON and setting it to a particular level – the Inputs of LOW, MEDIUM or HIGH -- results in a certain amount of heat, which is the Output. Transport is the process of transporting electric current from the wall socket into the heater, as well as the heat from the heating coils into the room. Conversion, represented by the heating coils, is what transforms the electrical energy into heat or thermal energy. The Structure element is the entire unit that contains all the components of the system.

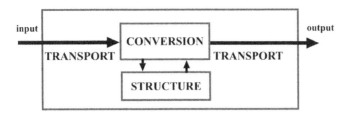

All open systems take in an Input and produce a specific Output. One underlying assumption of open systems is that the Output maintains itself as long as the Input is maintained. Human beings can also be open systems – and there's nothing wrong with that, if it's a conscious choice. The assumption is, for example, you show up to work, work hard and you get as Output a steady income, a stable relationship, and security --- all of which are worthwhile desires. They are certainly what most people hoped for and wanted during much of American history.

But now life is more fluid, unstable and improvisational. Change happens faster. It's no longer easy to even imagine what things were like before laptops and cellphones, even though they've only been around for a relatively short time.

So let's be clear about the relationship between the Input and Output in open systems. An open system provides for a stable and predictable result that is as close to being guaranteed as it can possibly be. If external disturbances occur that affect the result --- the Output --- open systems are not capable of self-correction or self-regulation to adjust the system in order to obtain the original Output.

And once again, there's nothing wrong with getting predictable results from well-understood and conventional actions, provided it's what you really want. But that's becoming more difficult in a world where rapid change is the norm. New technologies and historical changes are demanding that we be more flexible and resilient. For survival and success in that world, an open system existence might no longer be the best choice.

CHAPTER 15

Intelligent Systems

Intelligent systems include four additional elements: a Goal; Disturbances; a Sensor; and, a Controller. These elements enable self-regulation and continuous adjustment of the Input in order to achieve a desired Output that matches the Goal. Using a Sensor and a Controller, this can be achieved in spite of Disturbances to the system.

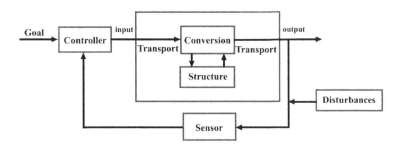

Unlike an open system, an intelligent system begins with a Goal, an intention, (or a *Dharma* or *Sankalpa* as they are referred to in Siddha). Setting this Goal is your responsibility and the Goal must be chosen wisely. The entire process of being "intelligent" exists to achieve that Goal, in spite of any Disturbances that occur.

Disturbances are those things that get in the way of achieving our Goal. They can be physical obstacles, or procrastination, inability to focus, and poor eating habits. In Siddha, obstacles were known as *vikaras*. The ancient Siddhars meticulously itemized all the known vikaras a human may face in a lifetime.

But, here is the secret: if we can use and refine our *Sensors* to know the current Output --- where we are at right now, and then use and develop our *Controller* to measure the difference between where we want to go --- our Goal and our Output to strategically figure out a new Input to affect the forces of Transport, Conversion and Storage to get a desired Output, we can move closer to our Goal. And, this process occurs over time as we go around the loop, and each time getting closer to our Goal.

We do this by "closing the loop" of the open system, by feeding back the Output of the open system to a Sensor, which is used to measure the actual Output. In the Siddha tradition, the Sensor was known as the *Indriyas* of the human body --- the Indriyas were our literal senses of smell, touch, sight, taste and hearing. How well the Sensor can measure is critical to knowing exactly where we are. A poor Sensor can give us an erroneous measure of the Output, and this will affect the decisions of the Controller. In Siddha, the purpose of awareness practices such as meditation, yoga and other spiritual activities was to enhance one's indriyas (sensors). The more our sensors are refined, the closer one can get to the Goal or Sankalpa.

The Controller (or *Manas* in Siddha) literally measures the difference between our Goal and the actual Output to make a decision on what new Input (or Karma) we need to send back into the system to affect changes in the forces of Transport (Vata), Conversion (Pitta) and Storage (Kapha), to get a new Output (Karma-Phal).

The Controller element is perhaps the most important aspect of intelligent systems. The Controller is all about making decisions. By integrating the Goal with information coming in from the Sensors, the Controller makes decisions which result in actions that are new Inputs into the system. These Inputs result in the Transport and Conversion of information, matter, and energy within a Structure, which leads to a new Output. As the sequence takes place and we become aware of the Output from our actions, the Controller draws on this awareness to make a subsequent decision. This results in a new Input. Based on that new Input, the process of Transport and Conversion of information, matter, and energy within a Structure is reiterated and refined.

When Disturbances are encountered, the system must course-correct back toward the Goal. Because this is a continuous process, it's critical that awareness and information – and the decisions that result – can be made on the fly. The more refined our awareness becomes by developing our Sensors, the better our decisions will be. For this reason, spiritual practices, which promote stillness and refinement of our awareness --- the Sensors, enable a clearer perception of what is really taking place and to see the Output with accuracy as it really is. This in turn allows the Controller to make better decisions. When in doubt, therefore, it's important to be still and refine your awareness.

Rather than a strictly spiritual approach, this is a principle of modern systems theory. It is also the essence of Siddha, which teaches stillness as a path to awareness, right decisions, and right action – which together result in the Output of achieving the Goal we desire. In both systems theory and Siddha, this process is what intelligence really means.

At any point in life, we can simply be reactive to what's happening around us, or we can set and approach our goals based on awareness, intention, and intelligence.

Every journey begins with a Goal and some level of awareness. As our awareness becomes more refined, our Controller can make decisions that translate the forces of information, matter, and energy into transport and conversion within a structure that leads toward the goal. The key lies in continuing the process of refining awareness and information, which may even lead to refining or redefining the Goal itself.

CHAPTER 16

An Intelligent System in Action

To make the concept of intelligent systems more real and practical, let's consider a home's central heating system that includes a thermostat. It's a good example of how an intelligent system works. Unlike the open system heater we discussed earlier, this "intelligent" system provides for constant refinement and adjustment of the Input to achieve an Output that matches a specific Goal.

Let's first identify the nine components of the intelligent system using the home heating system as a reference.

Goal: If the desired temperature for the apartment is 78 degrees, that's the Goal. It is achieved when the apartment's actual temperature (the Output) and the selected Goal are equal.

Disturbances: The opposite of a Goal, or the opposition to it, are Disturbances. In the thermostat example, the disturbances could be *a cold draft* from an open window in another room. Resolving Disturbances is the key to achieving the Goal. And, this requires accurate and refined Sensors as well as an effective Controller.

Sensor: The sensor is something that can measure the actual temperature in the room— *a thermometer* – within the thermostat. The Sensor communicates the actual room temperature (the Output) to the Controller. One thing to be aware of is that the sensitivity of the Sensor --- how refined it is in measuring the actual room temperature -- will be critical in achieving the goal of 75 degrees.

Controller: The Controller is the component of the thermostat that receives two pieces of information: 1) what the Goal is --- in this case 75 degrees, and 2) the actual room temperature from thermometer, which is the sensor. The Controller takes these two pieces of information and determines the difference between the Goal temperature and the current temperature.

Transport: The forces of Transport in this case are the flow of heating oil into the furnace. If our current temperature --- the Output --- is too low, say only 60 degrees, then the Input will be <u>to increase the transport (or flow)</u> of heating oil into the furnace. More heating oil, more heat. If this happens and the heat goes too high -- say to 80 degrees -- the Controller will send an Input to shut off the flow of heating oil into the furnace.

Conversion: The furnace takes in the heating oil (matter) and converts it into heat (thermal energy). The more oil, the more heat is produced. Less oil, less heat is produced. No oil, then no heat is produced. It's that simple.

Structure: The Structure is composed of the walls, the floors, the insulation, the beams, and the ceiling. These elements form the structure of the house, which provides a container where the forces of Transport and Conversion come together. Clearly, if you have very well insulated home, then the place will need much less oil to heat, and we can achieve and, more importantly, *maintain* the Goal --- with far less fluctuations. If the home has lots of drafts and poor insulation, heat will escape and the Controller will constantly have to turn on and turn off the flow of oil into the furnace.

Output: The Output is the actual temperature of the room at any point.

The key feature of intelligent systems is that they are always in flux. They are constantly making adjustments. They are sensing, controlling and modulating the input into the open system. "Perfection" is not the objective, but is only an imaginary concept, which is always being approached but is never permanently sustained.

CHAPTER 17

Systems Theory in the Kitchen

Perhaps the best way to understand systems theory is to see it in action in your everyday life. Suppose, for example, you wanted to make a few bowls of soup to serve to some friends on a chilly afternoon.

There are two ways of looking at this example. First, we can imagine making soup as an open system process.

It's very simple. Open a can of soup, put the soup in a pan, and turn on the stove for five minutes.

There are three Inputs: (1) opening the can of soup, (2) putting the soup in the bowl, and (3) turning on the stove for five minutes. The heat activates energies of Conversion to cook the soup. The pan provides the Structure. The Transport is the flow of heat energy through the pan and into the soup. After five minutes the Output is heated soup, which is ready to be consumed.

But suppose you were a more ambitious chef who wanted to make a large amount of soup using an intelligent system. What are the elements relative to the intelligent system of making soup?

Let's start with the Goal. We don't want just any bowl of soup. We want *a tasty, warm bowl of soup* --- this is our Goal. So far, so good.

But with any Goal, Disturbances will arise. There might be a power outage or an overflow of water. The kitchen might run out of a key ingredient. An important employee might suddenly quit in a huff. If something can go wrong, it often will. These are the potential Disturbances.

Remember, we achieve our Goal by overcoming Disturbances through the use of our Sensors and a Controller.

In this case, our five senses are the Sensors. We can observe how the soup is coming along by watching it. We can use our ears to hear if it boiling too much? Does something smell like it's burning? We can taste it so see if it has enough salt, or if it's too spicy or needs more sour taste. We can stir it and feel it with our hands to see if it's too thick or coarse. Our senses are fed back to our Controller.

The Controller is you, which includes your experience, your intelligence, and your skill as a chef. Are you getting closer to that tasty, warm bowl of soup? Based on this, you decide what action and inputs you are going to take and keep adjusting the inputs, until you achieve our Goal.

The Inputs could include adding or removal of ingredients, choosing to cover the pan, adding more salt, and increasing the flame.

Transport is the movement of heat and mechanical forces inside the pan, including the simple motion of moving heat as we stir the ingredients.

Next comes the energy of Conversion. The fire that heats the soup embodies this energy.

Structure is provided by the cauldron in which the ingredients are cooked and stirred.

The Goal is reached when, after continuously sensing the soup (tasting it, smelling it, touching it) and making adjustments with our Goal in mind, we get an Output, the tasty bowls of homemade soup.

PART 5

The Rosetta Stone and Beyond

CHAPTER 18

The Bridge Between Two Worlds

Following my doctoral work, I returned to India on a Fulbright grant. While in India, I made a discovery that transformed my life and how I look at the world. New foundations and breakthroughs in human knowledge emerge when disparate systems of knowledge and worlds are connected and unified, and that is exactly the kind of breakthrough I experienced. Technically speaking, I can describe it as identifying the systems theoretic basis of eastern medicine. But I prefer to think of it in more poetic terms, as the discovery of the scientific equivalent of the Rosetta Stone.

Years ago, when visiting the British Museum, I saw the Rosetta Stone on display behind a protective glass casing. It was an amazing experience to see this part of history: a big block of partially broken black and grey stone. The inscriptions on it were still visible. As I studied it, my memory pulled me back to my tenth grade European History class and the teacher who taught us how Napoleon's army in 1799 had unearthed the stone at their Fort Rosetta, during the invasion of Egypt.

Why was this stone important? Why was it protected and displayed with such reverence in the British Museum?

The discovery of the Rosetta Stone provided a gateway between two worlds: ancient and modern, east and west. Up until the time it was decoded, many scholars had difficulty in understanding hieroglyphics, the text used by the Egyptian civilization. While some hieroglyphics had been translated, the vast majority were still a mystery.

On the Rosetta Stone, carved around 190 BC, was a speech or decree by the council of priests, praising Ptolemy V, the new Greek King, recently been put into power as the king of Egypt. This decree was written in three languages side by side: hieroglyphics, an Egyptian script known as Demotic, and classical Greek. The writing on the Rosetta Stone made it possible for scholars to read the decree in three languages simultaneously. In this way, they were able to build a translation and open the door to an understanding of ancient Egyptian history. The stone served as a kind of thesaurus, or translator that provided a *lingua franca* or common language, which opened up the study of Egyptology by deciphering linguistic patterns across the worlds of ancient Egypt to Modern Greek.

In art and science, discoveries such as the Rosetta Stone are compelling not just because they bridge knowledge across the ages but because they interconnect disparate systems of knowledge to reveal a new understanding of existence. Interconnecting and integrating disparate systems reveals new truths that are bigger and different than the truths revealed by any one system alone. We all do this in our own way. And perhaps, the beauty of life lies in our common struggles to find such patterns of connection across the worlds we encounter.

Historically, there has always been a great divide, or even a direct conflict, between the Western scientific establishment and the traditions of Eastern medicine. Simply put, Western authorities felt they "knew it all," not only in the facts they had assembled, but also in the methods they had used to discover and categorize those facts. These methods, as we have discussed, were reductionist. They were hugely effective, as we have also discussed, but they were also limited -- more limited than Western science ever suspected.

While in India on my Fulbright grant, I realized that the principles of systems theory I learned at MIT was fundamentally analogous to the holistic principles of Siddha healing that I had seen my grandmother use. Western science, and especially medicine, was finally catching up with the anti-reductionist, fully integrated view of health and healing that had been the basis of Siddha for 5000 years.

This was truly the intellectual equivalent of the Rosetta Stone. It was the realization that Eastern and Western traditions could now be on the same plane, just as multiple languages, engraved on the Rosetta Stone, were saying the same thing. As I thought about this, I began to understand that even the metaphor of the

Rosetta Stone was inadequate to describe this emerging unity between East and West. This wasn't just the Rosetta Stone. It was the start of the Science of Everything.

CHAPTER 19

The Connective Tissue

Whether consciously or not, every man-made system, simple or complex, has been designed and developed based on the control systems engineering principles we discussed in Part Four. This is a basic principle of all reality. Since the human body is a complex system -- or even a system of systems -- systems biologists are adopting this principle in an effort to design and model complex inter- and intra-system interactions in the human system as a whole.

This approach is transforming biology from a purely experimental field into an engineering discipline. Without conscious awareness on the part of the innovators themselves, the principles of control systems engineering have already produced innovations that enhance the day-to-day lives of almost every human being. The thermostat in home heating systems, cruise control in automobiles, and the autopilot in aircrafts are examples of these innovations. Through a process of iterative understanding and modelling, systems of this kind are created and refined. The human system itself is a product of the principles of control systems engineering in which Nature, as the engineer, has refined and evolved the human system over billions of years.

Identification of the core principles of Control Systems Engineering, as well as itemization of the terminology used to describe those principles, are central components of The Science of Everything. These core principles of control systems engineering are derived from the notion of a system formalized in General Systems Theory, and from concepts of intelligent systems and closed systems based on feedback theory and linear system analysis that integrate concepts of network theory and communication theory.

General Systems Theory (GST) arose from disciplines including biology, mathematics, philosophy, and the social sciences. The Austrian biologist Karl Ludwig von Bertalanffy (1901 – 1972) began to formulate GST in the 1930s. However, his ideas did not receive widespread attention until much later. The aim of GST was to be a "unifying theoretical construct for all of the sciences." Another definition spoke of "a set of related definitions, assumptions, and propositions which deal with reality as an integrated hierarchy of organizations of matter and energy." In other words, a Science of Everything.

Western histories trace the origin of control systems engineering concepts to Greece in approximately 300 BC. These histories refer to the development of the water clock of Ktesibios, which used a float regulator that employed control systems engineering principles. But such histories seem unaware of the development of Siddha and Ayurveda, which were founded on the principles of control systems engineering.

This becomes evident when we juxtapose the terminology of modern control systems engineering with the terminology of Siddha and Ayurveda.

The Table below can be understood as a "Rosetta Stone," demonstrating that the foundations of the systems biology in Siddha and Ayurveda are the same as the principles of control systems engineering.

Control Systems Engineering	Siddha and Ayurveda
Input	Karma
Output	Karma-Phal
Transport	Vata
Conversion	Pitta
Storage	Kapha
Goal	Sankalpa
Controller	Manas
Sensor	Indriyas
Disturbances	Vikaras

This Table is the "Rosetta Stone" that connects Siddha with systems theory.

The terms Karma and Karma-Phal are the same as Input and Output of an open loop system. Vata, Pitta and Kapha are the same as the principles of Transport,

Conversion and Storage, which are central to modern systems theory and to Control Systems Engineering. Sankalpa is the Goal that one seeks to achieve. The Manas is the Controller that receives feedback from the Indriyas, which are the Sensor, to assess the current state of the system. Finally, the Vikaras are the Disturbances that are always present, which test the efficacy of a closed loop system to regulate its Input (or Karma) to achieve its particular Goal (or Sankalpa).

CHAPTER 20

Holism and Personalization

The systems biology of Siddha and Ayurveda provides two important features that today's modern Western systems biology seeks to replicate: first, *holism*, and secondly *personalization* within a framework of control systems engineering.

Siddha and Ayurveda developed a holistic understanding of existence from the immaterial to the whole human form. This holism provided a unified model of the whole, progressing from non-existence (Purusha) to material existence (Prakriti), leading to the materialization of subtle energies (Gunas), which then transformed to more grosser forms of matter (the Panchabuthas), that gave rise to a constitutive model called the Tri-Doshas. The three doshas, Vata, Pitta and Kapha, were central to defining the constitution of the body (Kosha), an individual's Prakriti, which affected the tissues (Dhatus) as well as the Kosha's organs, senses and mind.

The systems biology of Siddha and Ayurveda recognized fundamentally that health and well-being had to be personalized, and that there was no "magic bullet" solution, no one-size fits all. The concept of the individual Prakriti provides a mechanism to *personalize* care to find the right therapies that enable the individual to find an optimal state of health that may be very different for another individual. Moreover, there was a clear recognition that health was an ongoing and iterative process, where the individual needed to continually make refinements to their actions, based on sensory feedback from their environment and an intelligent assessment of the results of their actions.

As the Rosetta Stone reveals, the originators of Siddha and Ayurveda created an integrative framework that interconnected its nine concepts: Karma, Karma-Phal, Vata, Pitta, Kapha, Sankalpa, Manas, Indriyas, and Vikaras into a cohesive systems-based regulatory process, that enabled an individual or practitioner to use fundamental principles to manage health. Today, the western world refers to this same process as control systems engineering, conveyed simply in a different language: Input, Output, Transport, Conversion, Storage, Goal, Controller, Sensor and Disturbances.

To the best of my knowledge, this *Science of Everything,* which I first published as "The Control Systems Engineering Foundation of Traditional Indian Medicine: the Rosetta Stone for Siddha and Ayurveda" in the *International Journal of Systems of Systems Engineering,* is the first exposition demonstrating the connection between the core principles of Siddha and Ayurveda and their direct relationship to the concepts of Control Systems Engineering.

At a time when society is recognizing the need for alternatives to the current healthcare system, this Science of Everything provides a much-needed gateway across East and West, integrating ancient tradition and modern science. It provides a common language for understanding.

The ancient rishis and sages of India were not just men dressed in saffron robes but, at a fundamental level, were systems scientists. The irony is that many of the modern "gurus" have forgotten this origin, and today have created their own priesthood completely ignorant of the systems theoretic basis of Siddha and Ayurveda. They monetize this ignorance on multiple levels through their own reductionism giving tid bits of "holy" knowledge to their followers, who they enslave to some singular form of mediation, diet, yoga or ritual practices.

The Science of Everything, therefore, provides the gateway to not only for Western medicine to overcome its own reductionism and embrace Siddha from a solid scientific basis but also to liberate many who have been duped by the "gurus" and priesthood of the East.

PART 6

The System of Your Physical Self

CHAPTER 21

Your Body is an Intelligent System

Intelligent systems as we have seen are based on the desire to achieve a Goal. According to the traditional wisdom of Siddha, the body has a natural intelligence and it inherently knows its goal --- which is known as its *Prakriti* or its *Natural Systems State*. The Natural System State is the unique combination of the forces of Transport, Conversion and Structure inherent to you as an individual. In Siddha, health is defined as you achieving the goal of your body's Natural System State. Most of us are not even aware of our body's Natural System State. Disturbances, moreover, get in the way and perturb us away from our Natural System State.

Therefore, in Siddha the pathway to health begins by knowing our Natural System State – the goal, knowing how Disturbances have moved us away from this goal, and then making the adjustments through the inputs of food, exercise and supplements to bring us back to our Natural System State.

To begin: what is your natural systems state? In terms of systems theory, who is it that you really are? The forces of Transport, Conversion, and Structure affect all forms of matter, energy and information throughout nature. The strength of these forces varies from one life form to another. That strength also varies among individuals – including you -- within a given species.

The importance of these variations is being recognized by Western medicine as better diagnostic tools become available and as genome research reveals the individual character of human DNA. But the concept that every person's physiology is a system with an individualized balance of energies has existed for thousands of years. This became clear to me when I received a Fulbright grant that allowed me to return to India for study of the ancient health tradition known as Siddha.

The Siddhars used their own bodies as experimental laboratories to understand the interaction of three essential forces which they called Vata, Pitta, and Kapha.

As we've seen, it's surprising – or maybe it's not surprising – that the Siddha principles of Vata, Pitta, and Kapha are exact parallels of Transport, Conversion, and Structure. Perhaps systems theory is simply a new terminology for ancient traditional wisdom. Whether we see ourselves as combinations of Transport, Conversion, and Structure -- or of Vata, Pitta, and Kapha -- each of us is a shifting and individualized balance of these energies. It's a balance that needs to be continuously acknowledged, understood, and cared for.

As the forces of nature interact within each of us, some of us have more Transport, others are strongest in Conversion, and still others are dominated by Structure. There are even a few very individuals who have an almost equal presence of each. The varying proportion of these forces is one of the most essential ways in which we are different from each other.

Initially, you need to identify your own Natural System State. Once this has been done, the goal of supporting that state becomes possible. So what is your essential nature? Which forces give direction to your being?

Are you dominated by the force of Transport?

Transport expresses itself as sensitivity to variations in flow, mobility, and movement. If Transport is your dominant force and that force is too high, you may feel nervous and agitated. If it's too low, you could feel very lethargic or depressed. Transport is in charge of everything that moves and is kinetic in our bodies, including the flow of energy and information. Because of this, Transport is regarded as the primary force without which Conversion or Structure could not function.

When Transport is not functioning correctly, all the other forces can go awry.

- Are you extremely uncomfortable in cold weather?
- Do you often juggle several activities at once?
- Do you think and talk quickly?
- Do you prefer spontaneity over scheduling?
- Do you tend toward dry skin and hair?

116

- Are you naturally thin, and do you lose weight easily?
- Do you grasp new ideas quickly, but wish you could remember more of what you learn?
- Do you impulsively start working on projects without thinking them through?
- Do you sometimes skip meals or forget to eat?
- Are you basically optimistic and enthusiastic?

Are you dominated by the force of Conversion?

Conversion manifests as sensitivity to variations in physiological processes such as metabolism and digestion, as well as analytical thinking and decision-making. If the forces of Conversion are not functioning well, you can experience health and emotional problems associated with the inability to convert and transform elements of Matter, Energy and Information.

- Do you very strongly dislike hot weather?
- Are you detail oriented and exceptionally good at processing information and data?
- Do you think things through before taking action?
- Do you metabolize food quickly and efficiently?
- Do view competition as an enjoyable challenge?
- Does your weight fluctuate?
- Do you prefer to have meals on a set schedule?
- Do you become impatient with yourself or others?
- Do you enjoy turning ideas into applications?
- Are your eyes especially sensitive to sunlight?

Are you dominated by the force of Structure?

Structure is the principle of containment for matter, information, and energy. Men and women who are Structure dominant are naturally able to sustain and tolerate more than other people. Structure forces foster relaxation and calm, and an aura of security. But when Structure is out of balance it can manifest as stubbornness or isolation.

- Do you have a broad body frame?
- Do you tend to be overweight?
- Do you prefer not to move around or travel?
- Are you often called upon to help others?
- Are you not bothered by either hot or cold weather?
- Do you have exceptionally good physical stamina?
- Is your preferred learning style slow and steady?
- Do you easily retain what you've learned?
- Do you take your time moving between activities?
- Do you often have sinus infections or colds?
- Do you try to speak precisely and emphatically?

CHAPTER 22

Identifying Disturbances

Disturbances are part of any journey, including the journey of our lives. Once you become aware of your Natural System State, it's your responsibility to keep that state in balance, despite any turbulence you encounter.

But at any given moment you are likely not operating at the peak of your Natural System State. So how are you right now? How are you feeling today? Is everything going well in your life? Do you feel upbeat and cheerful or do you feel down in the dumps? Are you feeling healthy? Or are you catching a cold?

As a unique and dynamic person, you are not going to be feeling the same every day. Here are some questions to help you get a handle on what the forces of Transport, Conversion, and Structure are doing in your system, right now. Your answers will help you determine which forces are "off-course." You can then decide how you want to bring that force back into alignment.

Are your Transport forces undergoing disturbances?
- Have you been feeling anxious or overly excited?
- Is your energy level noticeably uneven?
- Are you feeling depressed, or do you have bursts of energy so intense that you have a hard time calming down?
- Do you have any dry spots, chapped, or cracked skin?
- Is your lower GI tract upset? Are you having bouts of diarrhea or constipation? Do you experience gas or bloating?
- Are you forgetting to eat, or are you losing weight?
- Is cold weather bothering you more than usual?
- Are you having difficulty concentrating or finishing projects?
- Are you having joint or arthritic pain?
- Have you been making any impulsive decisions?
- Do you have trouble falling asleep or staying asleep?

Are your Conversion forces undergoing disturbances?
- Are you putting pressure on yourself or others?
- Are you having upper GI problems?
- Are you suffering from heartburn or a sore throat that your doctor thinks is caused by acid reflux?
- Is an aversion to heat becoming more intense?
- Do you need stronger sunglasses than previously?
- Are you easily angered or often impatient?
- Have you become noticeably critical of others?

120

- Do you drink large amounts of water or other beverages?
- Do you have more rashes or cold sores than usual?
- Do you have feelings of jealousy or need to get even?

Are your Structure forces undergoing disturbances?
- Are you having sinusitis, allergies, or congestion?
- Are you able to keep your weight under control?
- Do you crave carbs, chocolate, or other sweets?
- Do you want to sleep all the time?
- Do you have a white coat on your tongue?
- Are you generally feeling lethargic and dull?
- Do you often procrastinate?
- Do you accumulate things you don't need?
- Are you finding it difficult make changes in your life?
- Do you respond to stress with hostility?

By learning which forces are disturbed, you can be the Controller, making adjustments to Inputs that will bring you back to your Natural System State. But the first step is to correctly assess what's wrong. What is the true nature of the disturbance? Be real. Don't look for an easy answer, neither in reductionist science nor in reassuring New Age mysticism.

CHAPTER 23

Dealing With Disturbances

When disturbances arise between where you are now and arriving at your goal, you'll need to make some adjustments. That means eliminating any imbalances that have destabilized the forces of Transport, Conversion and Structure, and optimizing those forces instead.

Optimizing the Forces of Transport. Transport is expressed through movement. When it's in balance, Transport presents itself as joy, grace, agility and enthusiasm. Both systems theory and Siddha identify three Inputs as essential for Transport to function at an optimal level: warmth, rhythm and lubrication.

Stay Warm
Our bodies, particularly our muscles, work far more efficiently when they are warmed up before any kind of activity or exercise. Muscles contract and relax faster when they are warm. Warmth gives your muscles greater

agility, speed, and strength. Warming up is like an insurance policy, decreasing the possibility of injury while also allowing you a greater degree of motion. If you are warm, your blood vessels are dilated, and this reduces stress on your heart and increases the flow (movement) of blood throughout your body. Blood is the key transporter of nutrients in your body. When you stay warm, your blood is able to be more efficient and deliver more oxygenated blood, making your entire system more effective to support motion at multiple levels. It also enables oxygen in your blood to be transported at a greater speed.

Your joints are key to movement and motion. Staying warm enables you to have a wide range of motion. Stiffness, for example, is a symptom that Transport is not working right. Warmth increases production of synovial fluids in your joints, serving to reduce friction, to support that range of motion. Greater range of motion gives you the greater confidence to try new things in a safe manner. Staying warm helps your body secrete the hormones that enable energy production, which is key to Transport. Exhaustion is another symptom telling us that the forces of Transport are not functioning right.

Movement can be erratic and chaotic, methodical and elegant, or graceful and intelligent. Staying warm enables nerve impulses to be transported at greater speeds, resulting in greater focus. This focus in turn will support the right level of concentration in a relaxed manner to provide support for graceful motion.

In order to thrive, Transport needs the Input of warmth. Think about your car on the coldest winter morning. Most of us will go out and warm it up before driving off. The warmth we are talking about is inner warmth, inside of the engine, inside of the car, inside of you. Warm friends, a warm home, and a warm disposition all fuel your inner forces of Transport. By doing those things that build such inner warmth, you directly support the optimal functioning of Transport.

Stay in Rhythm

A sense of rhythm is the ability to move your body to a regular beat. Rhythm or regularity is key to optimal motion and Transport. A person who dances well moves to a regular rhythm. A great drummer follows a great beat. Musicians often train with a metronome, an instrument that puts out a constant beat, to help them keep their rhythm. One of my mentors Frank Zane, the great body builder, taught me to lift weights to a metronome, or to a beat. When one does this, it makes it much easier, and more fluid. One can move and Transport with greater ease.

Because the force of Transport drives so many important body processes, it requires this level of regularity. Breathing, digestion and elimination are all dependent on proper rhythm and regularity. Having a regular schedule, eating at regular times, and sleeping and waking regularly is all about being in rhythm, which makes Transport far more effective. As someone said, "repetition is the mother of skill."

Siddha masters recommended that their students follow a schedule--early to bed, early to rise, routinized mealtimes, and play and work at particular hours. They were very demanding about the need for such regularity. In fact, in all spiritual practices, regularity is more important than the length of practice. Some people will meditate for 2 hours for a few weeks, and then stop, without any semblance of discipline. It is better to do less, but with consistency to achieve the best results. The highest level of rhythm and regularity is critical for the force of Transport.

In our breathing, the forces of Transport manifest themselves most clearly. Without breath our entire being ceases to exist. In the Bible, it is said that life began when God breathed into Adam's nostrils. The breath we have has a rhythm and regularity. That rhythm regularizes our pulse, our heart beat and our nerves. Emotions such as anger change our rhythm, and affect the forces of Transport. Every time we move or exercise, this is an exercise in breath. Breath is a gateway for us to see the force of Transport in action, and a way to measure our regularity moment to moment.

Stay Lubricated
Smooth and agile motion is supported by lubrication. All machines move better when they are well lubricated. Think about it. Your car will not move without oil and regular oil changes. Neither will you. To support Transport, your body needs to be well lubricated. Lubrication supports our joints, enables cellular motion,

lessens buildup of plaque in our arteries, and ensures that nerve impulses fire right.

Across a range of internal cellular processes, Transport needs lubrication. Without lubrication, the machinery of our bodies begin to squeak, get tight, rust, and motion stops. That squeaking door in your kitchen needs some oil. The stiffness in your joints would also benefit from some lubrication. Lubrication removes friction and ensures long-life of machinery, including your inner machinery.

The right kinds of oils and fats, and proper hydration support that lubrication. Wonderful research is being done and continues to be done on the value of different kinds of wholesome plant and animal based fats and oils. Doing your own research on them can prove to be invaluable. Healthy fats and oils play an overall role in supporting the forces of Transport. They contribute to an increase in energy and help us gain muscle mass. They also support the functioning of our heart, lungs, brain and digestive organs --- all components involved in Transport. The right lubrication makes our internal motors of motion that move air, blood, electrical signals run with ease and minimal friction. Healthy fats help protect our heart, an important motor-like pump, from cardiovascular diseases.

Our bones and skeletal structure keep us moving as we walk and run. Lubrication of the right kinds has been shown to strengthen bone density and reduce incidences of fractures, so as we age, we can still keep moving. Your skin is a major organ of transporting fluids and substances such as hormones, lymph, and water.

Hydration, which is a form of lubrication, is key to supporting movement of those fluids and substance to support the forces of Transport.

The right kind of lubrication supports internal cellular signaling, and the right signaling is key to cellular communication. Wrong communication results in illness and disease. Repeated studies have shown the value of lubrication at the cellular level to protect against various forms of cancer. Lubrication protects our machinery from rusting --- a process known in chemistry as oxidation.

That bicycle chain in your backyard has oxidized and is rusty. Put some oil on it, clean it up, and it's as good as new. Similarly, oils that are known as anti-oxidants can help remove the "rust" from our internal motors so Transport forces are able to glide smoothly. Nerve signaling, a type of cellular signaling, affects mood disorders. Stress affects nerve signaling and may result in increased depression and anxiety. The right kind lubrication increases levels of serotonin in the body. Serotonin makes people feel good and puts them in a relaxed state. Being relaxed supports agile Transport.

Optimizing the Forces of Conversion. The forces of Conversion are expressed as intensity and determination. When three key Inputs are present, Conversion presents itself as enterprising, brave, intelligent, ambitious, confident, and self-disciplined. These three Inputs are essential for Conversion to function at an optimal level: being cool, regulated and clean.

Stay Cool

Intensity doesn't need more intensity. Fighting fire with fire doesn't work here. The process of Conversion does the job of converting Matter, Energy and Information from one form into another. These processes all require "heat." However, in order to operate efficiently, they also need proper cooling.

A nuclear reactor, which is able to convert nuclear fission to thermal energy, is a classic example of Conversion. But a nuclear reactor needs those big cooling towers we see when pictures of reactors are shown. Your hot kitchen needs an exhaust system to keep it cool; your computer needs a fan to keep it cool.

Men and women with rapid metabolism and fiery dispositions – expressions of Conversion in action -- need to stay cool, in both mind and body, to balance their internal engines. Those with Conversion dominance need to look to the external world for ways to input cooling factors. This is different from those with a Transport dominance, who need to Input ways of increasing internal warmth.

Conversion dominant people need to avoid "hot situations" that can cause tempers to flare; they need to learn to "cool down" during those times when the intensity of action (during tough business negotiations for example) becomes too extreme. Staying Cool ensures that you don't overheat and burn up your internal engines, which are the power source of Conversion.

Warm-blooded animals sweat (like a human) or pant (like a dog) to dissipate heat through water evaporation. Sometimes it's easy just to cool off by going under a nice shaded tree or get some water on us. Other times it may be good just to take a vacation, "chill out" and go to cooler areas. Sometimes just sitting and watching the sunrise or sunset and other of Nature's beauty can serve to provide the cool to calm down and support the forces of Conversion, to remove the "heat."

Stay Regulated

The forces of Conversion are involved in the process of transformation and transduction. They convert energy from one form to another. The retina in your eyes convert light, electromagnetic radiation, to chemical impulses which are transduced to "see" the world. The engine in your car converts chemical energy to rotational mechanical energy.

This all involves many systematic and interconnected processes that need to be regulated correctly, with great sensitivity, to make sure that the inputs are converted to the right outputs.

If your retina does not transduce correctly, you get a blurred vision. If your car engine's pistons are not regulated with the right mixture of fuel and air to fire correctly, your car's motion could be accompanied by loud backfiring. All engines need to regulate their activity from action to rest, from focused work to regular maintenance --- in short they need to be in balance across the forces of motion and stillness.

Conversion can create a tendency to push too hard. They gravitate toward being on the go all the time, with extreme activity and little rest. If they don't learn how to regulate their activities, they run the risk of "burning up" and "burning out". Sometimes, this inability to regulate their own internal engines, results in an attempt to control everything, and everybody, in their environment. It would be better for them to learn how to control and regulate their own activities.

It can be difficult for a conversion dominant person to "let go" and relax with themselves and others. Their tongues can become harsh and mean --- an inappropriate way to control a situation, because in reality they are not able to control themselves. Extremes of this out-of-control behavior include throwing tantrums, becoming manipulative, all of which reflect a lack of self-regulation, which can backfire much like a car engine, whose internal pistons, misfire. High performance jet engines are designed to function well. They are able to operate across a wide range of temperatures and altitudes. They can regulate their engine performance across a variety of conditions, can adjust and adapt. Conversion forces require proper regulation to ensure their optimal functioning.

Regulation includes setting bounds of operation. Those who are dominated by Conversion forces can achieve great success if they are given, or create for themselves, internal and external boundaries. A high performance car also has its boundaries, if you "red-line" above a certain number of RPM's, the engine will conk out. The forces of Conversion operate well within their lower and upper bounds.

Work and rest are therefore equally important for these forces of Conversion. Forces of Conversion, like a motor can "be on" all the time, and not know when to stop. Men and women with strong Conversion forces have a tendency to overdo just about everything. They can work too hard, they can exercise too much, and they can over-do it with their attention to detail. Our Conversion dominant friends sometimes need to relax and stop competing. They need to learn to modulate their behavior, keeping everything more reasonable and moderate.

Regulating your behavior also implies being able to "surrender" and "go with flow" at appropriate times. Those with dominant Conversion forces can sometimes appear always to be on "high alert" in terms of a need to control the people and things in their environment. They need to learn how to regulate their behavior by stepping back and surrendering. It's essential to know when to stop, relax, rest, and shut down.

Stay Clean

Like any high performance engine, forces of Conversion thrive in a clean environment. This includes both high quality fuel and a clean internal mechanism. People dominated by Conversion need to be very careful about what they input into their bodies. Whole foods, organic and without preservatives and additives are wonderful because they provide "clean" fuel.

There is an emerging movement among pioneering food manufacturers in formalizing the definition of such clean foods through a newly developed Certified C.L.E.A.N. international standard, which I helped to facilitate using a systems-based approach that defines such foods as ones that have multiple attributes including being safe, non-GMO, organic, and having high bio-availability of nutrients. Keeping an eye out for such clean foods can serve to support Conversion.

Food combining is another wise strategy for ensuring effective transformation within our digestive systems. Slow-cooked foods, in many ways pre-digested, make it easy for our internal engine to absorb nutrients. In addition, regular and moderate fasts allow our engines to clean and heal themselves by supporting the body's own self-healing processes.

Optimizing the Forces of Structure. Structure brings stability, and stability is essential for survival. Men and women in whom Structure is dominant tend to have stability in their own lives and they like to provide it for others as well. The three Inputs that encourage Structure's optimal performance are: being dry, active and flexible.

Stay Dry

The force of Structure provides containment and support. When a home is built, the foundation represents the Structure force that holds the entire house. If the foundation (or basement) is damp or wet, the building's entire infrastructure is at risk.

Excessive dampness in your body's foundation can show up as cysts, tumors, chronic sinus infections, and yeast infections. Dryness can also have the benefit of slightly raising the body's temperature, creating a structural environment that is resistant to viruses and bacteria. A dry sauna, for example, can be ideal for supporting Structure.

Stay Active

Use it or lose it. Any physical structure, including the human body, gets stronger the more it gets used and stimulated. If you don't use your muscles, your skeletal structure, you atrophy. Structures that are not used are vulnerable to decay and rust. Various types of stimuli are critical in keeping a structure activated.

At the cellular level, the cell membrane and cytoskeleton, support the structure of the entire cell. Nature ensures that this structure is under constant stimuli to keep it vigilant and active so it supports the cell structure. Such activity increases the number of macrophages. Macrophages enhance the immune system and support structure by killing invading bacteria and viruses.

Physical activity also increases blood flow, allowing antibodies to move through your system and attack and remove bacteria and viruses. For those who suffer from inflammation, anti-inflammatory cytokines, which are the cell-to-cell signaling molecules, are themselves activated by physical activity. These molecules have a beneficial effect in promoting anti-inflammatory effects. This is one of the important benefits that come from being active because chronic inflammation causes most of the degenerative diseases such as cancer.

The forces of Structure provide framework and inertia. This inertia can also result at its extremes in laziness, moodiness, and immobility. Sometimes those

133

who are dominant in the forces of Structure "just don't feel like moving." Inertia and a lack of movement can contribute to a sense of depression or lethargy. Exercise and physical activity stimulates neurotransmitters in the brain to make one feel happier, less moody, and less depressed. Inertia is also implicated in osteoporosis, a structural disorder that causes bone loss. Exercise and physical activity is prescribed as a treatment for those who have osteoporosis or are in danger of getting it because it can help prevent and arrest the problem.

In order to hold things, Structure itself requires containment. The tendency to "holding on" often spells out issues with weight. Being active is a great controlling and modulating factor to manage one's weight. There is no better cure for the inertia and laziness of Structure forces than to boost one's energy level through physical activity. Diseases such as diabetes manifest when the forces of Structure go to its extremes of containment. Being active can be help deal with this condition. Activity helps makes the body more sensitive to insulin, to support burning of glucose e.g. calories. This helps to lower blood glucose and stop sugar spikes. Diabetics who exercise have been shown to need less insulin or medication than those who don't.

People with Structure dominance can also become too complacent and reliant on the status quo. They have a tendency to not want to "let go" of anything, including relationships and objects. They can "hold onto" relationships, situations, and things that no longer have value in their lives. Activity—getting out in the world, meeting new people, and trying new things—is a way of fighting this tendency.

Stay Flexible

Structure contains the elements of water and earth. Structures composed of water and earth can get stuck, muddy, swampy, and immobile. The most powerful structures in the world are not rigid, but flexible. If something is too hard, it can become brittle, and just shatter and break. In civil engineering, when larger structures are built, particularly in earthquake zones, they are designed to sway and to be flexible; sometimes they are even put on rollers, so they will move with the wave of the earthquake. The largest modern skyscrapers in the world now actually flex like pine grass in the wind.

This is a wonderful example of how flexibility can provide additional strength and make structures strong enough to withstand even the most powerful of Nature's forces. Similarly, flexibility is key for someone who is Structure dominant. If you become too stiff, you too can break or fall apart by life's continual and ongoing disturbances and changes. If you become too set in your ways, you might end up feeling as though you are stuck in a quagmire that resembles nothing so much as a muddy swamp.

Flexibility gives structures greater strength. Joints and fascia are particularly improved by flexibility. Blood flow can be increased by flexibility exercises such as stretching, which removes toxins and waste products that can cause a structure to "squeak" and get stiff.

Stretching the joints also results in improved blood flow, which, in turn, can cause slight increases in tissue temperature; this supports circulation and increases the flow of rich nutrients to the joints creating greater elasticity and higher levels of structural performance.

Flexibility allows structures to be more effective in dealing with environmental disturbances. My grandmother used to tell a story of two kinds of trees. One tree would bend when a river flooded and was able to go back to its original shape once the waters receded. The other tree would resist the flood and would ultimately be broken, ripped out from its roots. Structures that bend are more likely to survive.

Scientists have repeatedly shown how flexible structures can adjust themselves to reduce drag. It is clear that that unlike rigid structures for which an increase in velocity causes a squared increase of drag, the increase in drag for a flexible object is significantly lower.

Above all, it's your responsibility – and your opportunity – to become fully aware of the dominant energies of your being, and your Goal is to keep them in balance to support your Natural System State, not someone else's. Remember too that balance is not a passive state. It's achieved through strong action, and strong action is required to sustain it as well. There's a teaching by Vivekananda, one of India's contemporary spiritual masters, that alludes to this. Despite his metaphysical orientation, Vivekananda advised his students that if there was a choice between doing 50 pushups or meditating for 50 minutes, do the pushups!

PART 7

The Science of Everything at the Movies

Everyone's life is unique, yet all our lives have shared experiences. It occurred to me that watching movies is a shared experience for millions of people. And the content of many films, including some of the most successful ones, seem to very clearly use elements of systems theory. So discussing films as a way to illuminate systems theory seems like a good way to draw on an experience that millions of people have shared – that is, watching a movie.

The three films in this Part have been big successes critically and commercially. If you've seen them, I hope these discussions are revealing about the films as well as analogous events from real life. If you haven't seen them, perhaps now you'll be inspired to do as soon as possible for your own benefit. As the hero of *Gladiator* says, "What you do today will echo in eternity!"

CHAPTER 24

Gladiator

"A general of the Roman army is betrayed and becomes a slave and then a gladiator. And eventually he confronts the evil emperor who betrayed him in man-to-man combat."

This is how one of the characters in *Gladiator* summarizes the plot of the film. It's a good start but there's a lot more to say from a systems perspective.

Gladiator is the story of the Roman military commander Maximus, played by Russell Crowe. The film introduces Maximus as a citizen soldier who has left his farm, his wife, and their child in order to lead the Roman army. His deeply personal goal is simply to win the war against the barbarian hordes and return to his family.

But Maximus is also given a more public and political one by the dying emperor Marcus Aurelius. The emperor wants to designate Maximus as his heir in place of

Commodus, the emperor's corrupt son played by Joaquin Phoenix.

Commodus recognizes Maximus as a threat when Marcus Aurelius informs him of his intention to designate Maximus as his heir, thereby denying Commodus the possibility of becoming emperor.

Gladiator is an excellent resource for understanding the elements of systems theory and seeing how they play out in a complex narrative. Let's look at these elements one by one.

Goal: Commodus must be destroyed. This is Maximus' primary goal but – unlike Commodus' murder of Marcus Aurelius – Maximus does not simply kill his adversary even when he has the chance. Maximus knows that he must win the support and loyalty of the Roman people before real political change can take place. The balance of the film shows how Maximus gains that understanding and puts it into action.

Disturbances: In systems theory disturbances are the opposite of goals – the opposing energy. Commodus is Maximus' major disturbance. Systems theory includes two closely related elements that are basic to overcoming disturbances and responding effectively to them. These elements are the *sensor* and the *controller*. Just as disturbances are expressions of change, sensors and controllers are also dynamic in nature. They need to be upgraded from time to time as conditions change, and as you change during progress toward your goal.

Sensors: The sensors are those things that provide Maximus insight into what is going on so he can make decisions to guide him towards his goal. Early in the film, Maximus' sensors are not completely adequate to the hostile environment and the disturbances it presents. However, they provide unreliable intelligence. Later Maximus will come to rely and refine his own intuition and senses, even in the midst of being mortally wounded, to meet his goal.

Controller: Based on the information derived from sensors, a controller derives and implements a powerful action-oriented strategy. Initially when the gruff former gladiator Antonius Proximo purchases Maximus, as a slave, Maximus undergoes brutal training in Proximo's gladiatorial school. But Proximo soon becomes a mentor to Maximus. Specifically, Proximo once and for all diverts Maximus from a simple desire to kill Commodus for revenge. He makes it clear to Maximus that there is a larger issue that has to be addressed. Maximus has to be successful in the gladiatorial arena, and he needs to be entertaining while he does that. He has to win over the Roman crowd, because once they are on his side he can turn them against Commodus. This is the kind of insight a controller can provide.

Input: Inputs are the actions dictated by the decisions of the controller. In this case, they are the literal actions that Maximus takes to achieve his goal. Initially, Maximus knows that his actions must be congruent with everything that Proximo has taught him.

140

He has learned to fight well as a gladiator and win in the arena – and he must also gain the allegiance of the people by exciting and entertaining them. His actions are no longer about killing Commodus. It's about winning fights in the coliseum as a way to gain the final victory. Once Input is clear, the dynamic aspects of systems can manifest themselves. The foundations are in place, and meaningful action toward the goal expresses itself through the principles of *Transport, Conversion*, and *Structure*.

Transport: Transport is movement. In the early part of the film Maximus took some hard hits after being betrayed and sold into slavery. He becomes inert, depressed and lethargic. As Maximus interacts with Proximo and his comrades in the gladiator's school, he begins to move himself and eventually those around him as well. He reactivates the power of leadership that he showed in the film's early scenes as the general of the Roman army. He becomes an organizer and an inspiration to his fellow gladiators. He turns his fellow gladiators into a small, highly disciplined army – and he is once again ready to be a general and moves them into action towards his goal.

Conversion: Gladiator's fight scenes are the expression of the principle of conversion. Through each victory in the colosseum, Maximus converts the masses in the audience to become his loyal fans. Commodus challenges him to single combat in the arena. But the combat will be anything but fair. Commodus

141

treacherously wounds Maximus in the side just before the fight. Still, Maximus kills Commodus in the arena in a carefully choreographed action sequence. With his dying words, Maximus asks for the republic to be reinstated. The audience is converted to become loyal followers of his leadership, thereby enabling him to achieve his goal.

Structure: The coliseum and the crowd that populates it form the structural element of *Gladiator's* system. They are essential to the action, but they don't directly participate in it. The coliseum and the audience provide the structure within which the Transport (the movement) and Conversion (the fight) occur.

Output: Within the storyline of the film, *Gladiator's* Output is Maximus' winning over the audience to his side. The success of this Output helps Maximus assess whether he's heading towards his sacred goal – the restoration of the Roman republic. But it's interesting to note that the Output of the film exists in another form as well.

Whatever the goals of the characters in Gladiator may be, the movie itself is also a system with goals of its own. The film's goals include, first and foremost, the need to make a profit, and also to be artistically satisfying to the audience. Few movies are able to achieve both these objectives and Gladiator is one of the few.

CHAPTER 25

Apollo 13

Apollo 13 is a film based on a lunar space flight that was aborted when an emergency occurred on the spacecraft. The film was a commercial success and an even greater critical success. It received nine academy award nominations in 1995, winning in two technical categories. It won many other prizes as well.

Goal: Initially, the Goal of the Apollo 13 spaceflight is a landing on the moon. The astronauts will collect samples of moon rocks and bring them back to Earth. In the film's opening sequence astronaut Jim Lovell, played by Tom Hanks, hosts a party at his home to watch the first moon landing by Neil Armstrong. Lovell is scheduled for a moon flight – Apollo 14 -- but not until another crew goes to the moon first. We sense that his personal Goal is going to the moon, and his disappointment that he was not the first person to get there and that he will not be going to the moon for at least a year or more.

In the next scene, however, Lovell learns that he and his two companion astronauts – Ken Mattingly (Gary Sinise) and Fred Haise (Bill Paxton) – have been moved up to become the crew of Apollo 13. At this point the Goal of the film as a whole and Jim Lovell's personal Goal become one and the same. It's all about making Apollo 13 a successful flight to the moon.

Disturbances: It's just one thing after another. From the first moment until the last, *Apollo 13* shows unexpected problems appearing. Most of them are of a technical nature, involving the operation of the rocket, the ability to complete the mission, or even to survive Disturbances like a breakdown in the oxygen supply or the extreme heat of reentry to the Earth's atmosphere. There are also interpersonal disturbances among the characters, both those in the rocket and on the ground in the mission control site.

Sensors: Just as there are lots of Disturbances in *Apollo 13*, there are plenty of sensors. In fact, there is a large room full of hard-working nerds in the mission control facility who are dedicated to keeping track of everything that happens on the flight and to identifying anything that goes wrong. Since plenty of things do go wrong, the sensors have an important role in the film. Some of them are grouchy, some of them are charmingly insightful, but they're all totally dedicated and extremely competent. They make us proud of them.

Even the dials and gauges in the rocket's cockpit – sensors in a literal way – play dramatic roles when, for example, they indicate the temperature inside the module or rising levels of life-threatening carbon dioxide. The Sensor gauges are our friends and advocates, just like the nerds back in Houston.

Controller: Apollo 13 is definitely a Controller's movie. Jim Lovell, of course, is a Controller in his role as commanding officer of the mission. But the most prominent Controller in the film is Flight Director Gene Kranz, played by Ed Harris, who supervises the technicians in the Mission Control Center. Kranz is probably one of the clearest personifications of a Sensor in any movie ever made.

Input: The character of Gene Kranz creates a strategy for the mission that has become the film's signature line of dialogue: "Failure is not an option!" At one point he challenges the technicians to fit a square piece of equipment into a round container: in other words, to put a square peg into a round hole. And they do it too. We don't see exactly how they do it, but we know that the software that Kranz downloads into the move is going to work, because failure is not an option. He does something like this many times during *Apollo 13*. We never find out how he does it, or what his experience and credentials are, but Ed Harris makes it perfectly believable.

Transport: This is the kinetic element of the film. It's all the scenes in which action is happening and movement taking place. Certainly there are images that obviously provide this component. The sequence of the rocket's fiery takeoff, the sequence in which the module flies low above the moon's surface, and the reentry of the vehicle through the Earth's atmosphere are a few examples. The whole movie is a mixture of the claustrophobic environment of the rocket and the Mission Control Center, and the infinite vastness of outer space.

Conversion: When the lunar module starts its descent to Earth, the three-man crew has learned to work perfectly together through the many Disturbances that have arisen.

Structure: The physical settings of Apollo 13 are unusually important, perhaps because there are so few of them. They mean a lot to us as viewers because they play a direct role in the action. We come to feel at home in the mission control center and the lunar module, especially when the characters go for days without shaving or sleeping.

Output: The Goal was not attained – but as sometimes (or often) happens the original goal was adjusted or even replaced. We see these adjustments happening all through Apollo 13, and the ability of the characters to respond to them is another thing we're urged to admire. The whole meaning of *Apollo 13* can be summed up in phrases like "things always happen for a reason" or "things turn out for the best." That such a successful film could be built on those kinds of sayings is testimony to the power of systems theory, at least when it's applied by very talented people.

CHAPTER 26

Joy

Joy is a very different kind of film from *Gladiator* and *Apollo 13*. In the language of Hollywood, Joy is what's called a "women's picture." The lead role and the principal supporting roles are played by women, and the primary audience for the film is also female.

Gladiator shows us the hero, Maximus, learning to fight in the arena. We see Russell Crowe, a major star, being instructed and upbraided by his mentor, Proximo. These scenes fulfill one of the anthropologist Joseph Campbell's major criteria for the development of an epic hero. That is, the hero must descend to the depths. He must seem to lose his heroic stature. In this way, he can rise again to greater heights than ever before.

An updated, female version of this happens in Joy. Instead of Russell Crowe being treated like a slave, we see Jennifer Lawrence – currently the premier actress of her generation – cleaning up spilled juice and demonstrating a mop in the parking lot of a KMart store.

Jennifer Lawrence hits bottom, and then rises to the financial heights. But instead of restoring the Roman republic or flying to the moon in a rocket, she gets rich by inventing a new kind of mop.

Goal: Joy Mangano (Jennifer Lawrence) was a precocious, extremely imaginative child who did very well in school. She loved to give form to her ideas by building models and acting out fantasies. But now, after marrying a failed lounge singer and having two children, she's trapped in a tedious job. She also lives in a house with her extended family of quirky relatives who are alternately funny and obnoxious, and who are closer to poor than rich.

Joy's personal, internal goal is to recapture the excitement and imagination of her childhood. In fact, we see a dream sequence in which Joy's own childhood self appears and makes that goal clear to her.

Joy's external goal is to get herself and her family out of their financial problems. After showing us Joy's predicament in the first twenty minutes of the film, we watch Joy have an epiphany when a glass of wine is spilled on the teak wood deck of a wealthy woman's yacht. At that moment, with her instincts as a creative engineer, Joy has an idea for a revolutionary mop design. The rest of the film depicts the twisting path toward the realization of her goals.

Disturbances: Joy is a creative and entrepreneurial woman but she's held back by her domestic situation. Her crazy family members aren't exactly happy with living hand to mouth in a crowded house, but it's what they're used to. They've developed so-called coping mechanisms. Joy's mother spends all day in bed watching soap operas. Her husband stays in the basement practicing his singing. Her sister has developed a personality based on humiliating Joy. Her father runs an auto parts company that barely stays afloat.

At the start of the film, these are Joy's Disturbances. More specifically, they're her distractions. They keep her disconnected from her true talents. As she begins to break free, new Disturbances crop up that are more than just distracting. But within *Joy* as a system, living uncomfortably in a crowded house is seen as really, really awful. It may even be worse than death, because there's nothing grand about it. It's low comedy rather than high tragedy.

Sensors: One of Joy's biggest problems early in the film is the complete absence of reliable Sensors. Surrounded by dysfunctional people who deeply misunderstand the real world, Joy's own perceptions are numbed by trying to keep the whole thing afloat.

Joy may not live completely in a dream world like her mother watching soap operas, but she is not seeing things clearly at the start of the film, and there is no one around who is seeing things clearly. But by the end of the movie she's become a really sharp businesswoman.

Controller: Joy eventually meets an executive at a TV home shopping network who becomes somewhat of a mentor to her, though not as central to the plot as was

Proximo in *Gladiator*. The executive, Neil Walker (played by handsome Bradley Cooper), inspires and instructs Joy about marketing her product on television. Walker is the controller in *Joy*. He directs her in selling her mops just as Ed Harris directed Tom Hanks in flying to the moon.

Input: Neil Walker instructs Joy to "be herself" when she appears on the television home shopping network. He doesn't tell her exactly what that means, but he inspires her to figure it out for herself and trust her instincts.

Transport: Since it's a film about making and selling mops, the director had to be creative in order to depict this in a kinetic, cinematic manner. It must have demanded rather more imagination than filming either a rocket taking off or a swordfight in a Roman arena. The film also uses the musical soundtrack in order to bring movement onto the screen. Mop manufacturing is accompanied by loud rock and roll.

Conversion: When Joy successfully markets her mop on television, the effect of the scene within the context of the movie is the same as Maximus fighting in the arena or Jim Lovell descending to Earth in a fiery re-entry vehicle. It's the culmination of everything that's happened up to that point. A similar effect is achieved at the end of the film when Joy confronts the crooked businessman in Texas who has tried to defraud her. But by then Jennifer Lawrence doesn't have to do anything to express Conversion except calmly look out of a window.

Structure: The action of Joy – family members yelling at each other, mops being made, mops being sold on television – takes place within convincingly rendered environments of squalor and sleaze. A stuffed fish on the wall of an unscrupulous, low-level businessman. A messy basement. A K-Mart parking lot. The structure of the film is decidedly unromantic or unglamorous. But the message is still that magic can happen here. You may not fall in love, but that's not what you really want anyway. You can make a lot of money.

Output: Joy's inner and outer goals are attained, and without the tragic conclusion of *Gladiator* or the bittersweet ending of *Apollo 13*. Joy is rich, and if she's emotionally alone not much attention is paid to that. She's also generous. When entrepreneurs like her former self appear in her office, she's glad to help them out. She's reached a high level of consciousness not just because she's succeeded, but because she's worked through all the Disturbances that arose without becoming corrupted.

Made in the USA
Monee, IL
22 August 2023

41443980R00085